THE CANCER TERMINATOR

Live stories of

100 cancer sufferers.

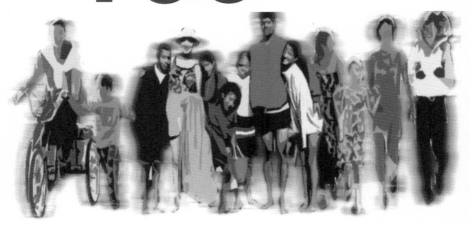

The Cancer Terminator

Live stories of 100 cancer sufferers

Editor:Wang Zhen Guo

Superisor:International Rehabilitation of Cancer

Published by:Chow Hoi Tong Cultural Enterprise

Publisher:Tai Cheuk Yin

Address:Rm.1607,Pacific Plaza,

418 Des Voeux Road West,Hong Kong

Tel:852-25415435

Fax:852-25415445

E-Mail:chowht@hkstar.com

Distributor:Chow Hoi Tong Cultural Enterprise

ISBN:962-542-017-7

First Edition: June 2001

Unit Price:HK$100

Japanese Edition:

First Edition:published in March 2000

Chinese Edition:

First Edition:published in Hong Kong in March 2001

English Edition:

First Edition:published in Hong Kong in June 2001

CONTENTS
Contents

Part 1

Chapter I

Traditional Chinese Medicine:
An Effective Treatment for Cancer?

Is Cancer really incurable?

Current situation of cancer treatment

The complementary functions of Chinese and Western Medicine

Characteristics of Chinese Traditional Medicine

Integration of Western and Chinese Medicine

Current situation of integration of Chinese and Western medical remedy

Chapter II

"Tian Xian Liquid"-
Traditional Chinese Anticancer Medicine

Traditional Chinese Medicine rerecognized by the Chinese government

The development of Tian Xian Liquid

Main contents and constituents

The Chang Bai Mountain -- "Treasure house of crude drugs"

Pharmaceutical actions of main crude drugs

Chapter III
·· 63

The effectiveness of treatments and precautions

From capsule to medicine liquid

To Improve the Quality

The Praises are Pouring in

The Characteristics of the Improved of No.1 Tianxian liquid

The Characteristics of the More Effective of No.1 Tianxian Liquid

The Characteristics of the No.1 Tianxian Pellets

The characteristics of No.1 Tianxian Suppositorium of China

The characteristics of No.1 Tianxian Plaster in China

Chapter IV
·· 85

The clinical experiments prove the effectiveness

The clinical experiments of ten research institutions

The anticancer medicine with extensive usages

(I) The experiments of animal toxicology

(II) The function of cell toxicity

(III) The influence to the cell period and DNA compounding

(IV) The strengthening effectiveness to radiation treatment

(V) The restraining function to the testing tumors

(VI) The dates of the clinical cases in the cancer treatment

Chapter V
How to Prevent Cancer and Cancer Transfer

Appendix

Part 2

One hundred cancer survivors' heart-warming
and amazing stories

Experiences of defeating uterus cancer
and breast cancer successfully

Experiences of defeating
breast cancer successfully

Experiences of defeating lung cancer successfully

Experiences of defeating liver cancer successfully

Experiences of defeating stomach cancer successfully

Experiences of defeating skin cancer

Experiences of defeating bone cancer

Experiences of defeating laryngopharyns cancer successfully

Experiences of defeating thyroid gland successfully

Experiences of defeating nose cancer successfully

Experiences of defeating esophagus cancer successfully

Experiences of defeating other diseases successfully

PART 1

Traditional Chinese Medicine

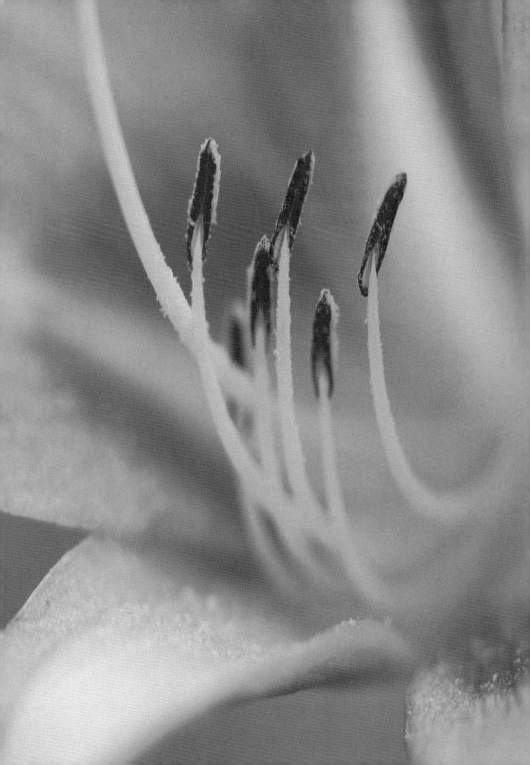

Chapter I

Traditional Chinese Medicine: An Effective Treatment for Cancer?

Is Cancer really incurable?

Many people believe cancer is incurable, and a patient who is suffering from this disease often being seen as a dying man.

In fact, cancer has been a cold-blooded killer for the humankind, depriving so many people of their precious lives. Though doctors have been trying their best to fight with it ever since the beginning of the 20th century, they are only frustrated to find their inability to come up with a miraculous cure. However, with the great leaps in medicine and developments of technology, doctors are now showing more confidence in coping with this herald of Azrael.

Cancer is difficult to defeat because the cancer cells are too gingerly and fast in spreading their territory. A doctor's failure to discover it in the early stage and once a diagnosis is confirmed usually it would be "too late" and no effective way of healing could be assured. Moreover, the origin of cancer and the mechanism behind it is still a mystery, not all cancers are therefore curable.

Nevertheless, there are numerous people fight against cancer and ultimately survive the battle. Patients suffered from the first phrase of such cancers as uterus, breast, stomach, esophagus, and laryngopharynx, the curable rate is over 90%. Even for the unluckiest people who are down with liver cancer, they can still live for five years longer. In effect, the discovery and treatment of the killing monster in its formative days will prove to be a successful measure to prevent it from devouring the unfortunate sufferer. Currently, medical experts across the world persist on the study of cancer day and night to seek for new discovery.　Unfortunately, over a sustained period of application of new inventions to the treatment, other unexpected side effect will arise, which place the doctors in a dilemma. As a consequence, new discoveries and new opportunities also turn out to be challenges to the doctors' intelligence.

Current situation of cancer treatment

At present, there exist a variety of treatments to cancer. Set out are brief introductions of some most representative treatments.

1.Surgical treatment.

In the early stage, the removal of the cancer nidus by surgery was the most effective way of treatment, not only the most orthodox, but also one of the most effective treatments. Full recuperation, of early cancer in particular, can be achieved nearly without exception by surgery. In case the cancer cells transfer to other parts, direct symptoms arising from the cancer can still be removed by surgery.

However, there still exist restrictions of the surgical method. The partial resection in any degree of the human body by surgery will inevitably render new injury. As normal organizations are cut apart and blood vessels, lymph and neural are cut off during the course of operation. Sometimes even more serious sequel will occur. Furthermore, provided the cancer cells have already intruded into vital internal organs or blood vessel lymph, the medical crew must take the safety issue of the operation into consideration.

In recent years, the laser or entoptic mirror method of resection has attracted much attention in the medical sector, not only enjoys a high success rate but also reduces the body injury and the rate of complicating disease. Therefore, the selection of the proper method is subject to the prudent appraisal of the medical group.

2.Anti-Cancer drugs treatment

The using of anti-cancer drugs is most effective in the treatment of leukemia and malignant lymphoma. In addition, it is also applicable to elimination of the cancer cells unable to be completely removed by operation, to the prevention of transference as well as the recurrence. However, with the employment of anti-cancer drugs, normal cells will be destroyed too together with the cancer cells and side effect will follow. Once the digesting, hematopoietic and lymphoid systems are destroyed, and due to the declination of white blood cell, anorexia, loss of appetite and inability of food intake, the physical strength will further decline. On the contrary to purpose of healing of the disease, due to incomplete metabolism and the consequent accumulation of the drugs within the body, cachexia will occur if it exceeds the loading range of human body.

General common side effects of the anti-cancer drugs include:

Inhibition of the bone marrow functions: due to the decrease of white blood cells, blood platelet, red blood cell, hemoglobin, the immunity will decline and consequently such symptoms as bacteria infection, fever, bleeding, lassitude will occur.

Declination of enterogastrocele function: thirsty, anorexia, nausea, vomitus, and inflammation of mucous membrane of mouth, ulcer, constipation, diarrhea, hemorrhage of gastrointestinal tract, abdominal pain.

Attenuation of immunity: incapable of identifying normal cells from abnormal ones, and even incapable of inhibiting the growth of cancer cells remaining within the body. Therefore, transference and recurrence are very likely to occur.

Attenuation of kidney function: backache and aching pain of lumbus, hematuria, edema, abnormity of urinary test, etc.

Attenuation of the liver function: liver pain, emergence of jaundice.

Attenuation of heart function: dilatation of heart, puffiness of limbs and face caused by disturbance of blood circulation.

Attenuation of lung function: intermittent hepatitis, over inflation of lung, fever, cough, expiratory dyspnea, etc.

Influence on neural: paralysis of hands and feet, abnormal feelings arising from peripheral neuritis.

Baldness: due to baldness, emotions will be affected; when in depression, free radical will be activated leading to the increase of cancer cells.

3.Radiotherapy

Radioactive rays inflict excellent casualties on the young cells with prosperous proliferation. They can completely destroy cell growth and can apply to the partial treatment. Likewise, they can kill cancer cells in proliferation or in transference to other part of the body as well as eliminate other cancer cells that cannot be completely removed by operation.

However, although radioactive rays can completely spoil cancer cells, normal cells simultaneously suffer from destruction. Therefore, for the patients with final phase cancer in extremely fragile health condition, the senior or patients with other chronic diseases, it would be inappropriate to apply radiotherapy on them.

Set out is the side effects of radiotherapy:

Sense of latitude, headache, vertigo, attenuation of immunity, etc.

Anorexia, nausea, vomitus, maldigestion, abdominal distension, and diarrhea, etc.

Decrease of white blood cell and blood platelet arising from the effect of inhibiting the production of bone marrow and the consequent hematopoietic disorder.

Possible symptoms of other part of the body:

Skin symptoms: flushing, itching, baldness, pigment precipitation, ulceration, congestion and edema, blister, and ulcer, etc.

Symptoms of the mouth cavity: inflammation of mucous membrane of mouth, thirst, alteration or complete deprivation of taste and smell senses caused by atrophy of salivary gland.

Symptoms of the brain: encephalatrophy, brain necrosis, myelitis, and disturbance of feelings and movement.

Symptoms of the lung: pneumonia, cough, expectoration, and fever.

The complementary functions of Chinese and Western Medicine

As all of the above-stated treatments are rooted in the western medicine, Chinese medicine would be a blessing for its long history of 5000 years and its function in repairing of the harms resulted from western medicine. There

Table 1 Current situation of the effect of anticancer agents

Effect Group	Treatment	Extended longevity	Tumor shrinking	Types of cancer
1	○	○	○	Acute lymphemia Most popular cancer of children
2	△	○	○	Breast cancer,Small-cell carcinoma of lung
3	✕	△	○	Stomach cancerNon small cell carcinoma of lungCervical cancerCervix cancerLarge intestine cancer
4	✕	✕	✕	Liver cancer Pancreatic cancer Hypothyroid cancer Stomach cancer

○: effective △: inconspicuous ✕: indistinguishable

(quoted from Daily News, November 12, 1995 『Consultation 5 of Anticancer Agent』.)

If western medicine defined as partial treatment, then Chinese medicine shall be defined as overall treatment. Only with the artful integration of both can we effectively fight against cancer.

remain a considerable number of records concerning pathogeny logics, subjective symptoms, and disease features appearing on the human body, and treatments, etc. in Chinese ancient documents. Many cancer-related records, in particular, were embraced in these documents. For example, "Regularity and Irregularity Doctrine", "Dialog on Medicine" both fall into the pathogeny theory of cancer as well as the conclusion drawn from effective treatments. They contain detailed records of theories and methods that even nowadays we still can follow. We will provide detailed introductions later in this book.

Chinese medicine enjoys the fame of "essence of clinical experience over thousands of years", which was achieved through practice and testing but in no sense hypothesis or deduction. Distinguished from the gents employed in western medicine, Chinese medicine boasts special therapeutical effects, which can be complementary to the insufficiency of western medicine in the above situation and thus provide an overall healing effect on cancer.

In fact, most Chinese traditional medicine possesses the functions to fight against cancer. For example, the ingredients of current anti-cancer drugs all come form natural plants and belong to the effective contents of Chinese medicine. They can directly or indirectly kill the cancer cells. In addition, Chinese medicine is especially renowned for its nutritional value and tonic effects through activating the immunity of the human body; once the immunity was enhanced, the body itself can inhibit, if not destroy the production of cancer cells. As a consequence, it is certain that the healing effects will be improved by the combining use of Chinese medicine, anti-cancer drugs and radiotherapy. It is also conducive to the recovery of the body energy after surgery.

Characteristics of Chinese Traditional Medicine

As delineated above, different approaches as Chinese and Western Medicine employ, they share a common target. As Chinese medicine boasts special theories and features, just like the treatments of cancer, there exist a considerable number of divergences between Chinese and Western medicine. Simply speaking, the advantages of Chinese medicine right correspond to the disadvantages of Western medicine. Set out is the brief introduction of the medical orientation of Chinese traditional medicine.

(1). Concept of wholism

From an integral perspective, Chinese medicine takes the whole body into consideration when treating illness. Since nidus affects the whole body, Chinese medicine not only pays attention to the therapeutical treatment of the nidus itself, but also stresses the enhancement of the immunity as a whole. With regard to cancer, Chinese medicine advocates that above all, it is necessary to remove the nidus to prevent it from further multiplication, proliferation, and transference so as to guard against deterioration and improve the immunity against cancer.

(2). Vital vs. Malignant Doctrine

All of the pathogens in Chinese medicine are entitled "malignant" while the resistance against diseases within the body is entitled "vital". Other than spiritual pressure that induces pathogen of cancer, there still exist other reasons, for example, stagnation of qi (a morbid condition due to impeded circulation of qi that leads to a local obstruction), blood stasis (a morbid state of blood stagnancy in a certain area of the body caused by sluggish flow of qi or blood and trauma), noxious heat (pathogenic and noxious qi), dampness accumulation (accumulation of pathogenic dampness), and accumulation of phlegm (a morbid state marked by impeded circulation of qi and blood, and phlegm remain in a certain area of the body), etc.

As cancer always arises from the insufficiency of vital qi and the malignant qi will take the chance of intrusion. Consequently, the phenomenon of "over accumulation and overlapping" occurs. The vital qi is constituted of such four elements as qi, blood, yin and yang. In case of the lack of sufficient vital qi, part of, if not the whole organs of the body start to enervate.

In the so-called stage of "pre-ailment" of the Chinese medicine, the most important approach of prevention from cancer is to maintain resistance and further accumulate vital qi. An Chinese saying "malignance withdraws in face of the vital qi" vividly interprets this. The occurrence of cancer can be compared to the combat between vital and malignant qi. In case the vital qi recovers and turns increasingly stronger, the malignant qi will enervate and, as a result, the state of illness will improve. Contrarily, provided malignant qi grows increasingly stronger while the vital qi fades, the state will deteriorate and consequently be driven into the last ditch.

(3). Comprehensive diagnosis

(diagnosis and treatment based on overall analysis of symptoms and signs, the cause, nature and location of the illness and the patient's physical condition according to the basic theories of traditional Chinese medicine)

Another unique feature of Chinese medicine lies on the affirmation of "syndrome" (a term to summarize collectively certain symptoms and signs according to the theories of traditional Chinese medicine). In simple words, different positions of cancer and different degree of deterioration lead to different syndrome. Therefore, "comprehensive diagnosis" turns out to be one of the most distinctive features of Chinese medicine for its efficient prescription fitting special state of illness.

The comprehensive diagnosis includes: the eight principal syndromes (serving as guidelines in diagnosis, namely, yin and yang, exterior and interior, cold and heat, deficient and excessive syndromes); differentiation of diseases according to pathological changes of the viscera and their interrelations; differentiation of syndromes according to the state of qi and blood; analyzing and differentiating of febrile diseases in accordance with the theory of the six channels (namely, the Taitin, Shaoyin, Jueyin, Yangming, Taiyang, and Shaoyang channels); and differentiation of syndrome according to the pathological changes of tri-jiao (including upper-, middle-, and lower-jiao, the upper of which houses the heart and lung; the middle of which, the spleen and stomach; the lower of which, the liver, kidney, urinary bladder, small and large intestines). The treatment of cancer mainly refers to three items as the eight principal syndromes, differentiation of diseases according to pathological changes of the viscera and their inter-relations; and differentiation of syndromes according to the state of qi and blood. The principle of "strengthening the body resistance to eliminate pathogenic factors" generally includes: hemostasis by invigorating qi(treating hemorrhage due to deficiency of qi mainly with drugs); nourishing yin and supplementing yang, clearing away heat and toxic material, regulating the circulation of qi (a therapy by using medicines which can promote the flow of qi, check its upward adverse flow, and replenish it to treat stagnation, adverse flow and deficiency of qi), promoting blood circulation by removing blood stasis, removing dampness and phlegm, resolving the hard lumps, softening and resolving hard mass (a therapy for masses formed by accumulation of phlegm and blood stasis); treating the toxifying disease with poisonous agents, etc. With reference to these principles, we can diagnose the cancer and work out specific remedies together with the appropriate selection of medical materials to soothe, if not cure it.

37

(4). Function adjustment

Chinese medicine enjoys stable and mild therapeutical efficacy with the prominent feature of slight side effect. Western medicine, in sprite of its acrid effects, brings about even acrid side effects, which plagued the West for a sustained period of time. Inevitably, there also exist side effect of Chinese medicine. However, it is likely to restrain it to the minimum with proper assortment of medical ingredients. Rather than merely help western medicine improve therapeutical efficacy of cancer treatment, Chinese medicine plays a more important role in the enhancement of the whole immunity of human body.

Integration of Western and Chinese Medicine

Generally speaking, Chinese and Western Medicine have their respective pros and cons. Western medicine, with the employment of operation, anticancer agents, and radioactive rays, emphasizes on the radical cure of cancer, which cannot be achieved by Chinese medicine. However, when we are keen on the strong therapeutical efficacy of western medicine, we shall not ignore their serious side effect. In this respect, the stable and mild Chinese medicine only renders slight side effect. Accordingly, there would be nothing better than the integral employment of Western and Chinese medicine, learning from each other's strong points to offset weaknesses. The Western remedy attacks cancer cells while the Chinese remedy offsets side effect as well as enhances the whole immunity of the human body. In this way, we can not only upgrade therapeutical efficacy, but also prevent from transference and recurrence. We will never be afraid of facing cancer anymore.

If western medicine is defined as partial treatment, then Chinese medicine overall treatment. Only with the skillful integration of both can we effectively fight against cancer.

If western medicine defined as partial treatment, then Chinese medicine shall be defined as overall treatment. Only with the artful integration of both can we effectively fight against cancer.

Current situation of integration of Chinese and Western medical remedy

The so-called integration of Chinese and Western medical remedy does not simply refer to the dual application of both Chinese and Western medicine, or adopt the other approach after a sustained period of employment of one. Above all, the conclusion of the respective advantages of the Chinese and Western medicine should be based on the analysis of the conditions as well as of the pathological features of the illness. With the tailor-made treatment scheme, it is likely to achieve the purpose of integrity, thoughtfulness and being well founded. Sets out are the specific approaches of combination:

(1). Treatment according to differentiation of symptoms and signs VS. Differentiation of illness

According to the western diagnosis of the illness, classification and TNM by stages, different treatment scheme can be selected from surgery, radiotherapy and anticancer agents. Then taking the analysis of the state of illness in different stages of Chinese medicine into condition, we can apply the treatment according to differentiation of symptoms. For illnesses of the same diagnosis results, due to the difference of one or two conditions or in different stages of the illness, the "syndromes" will vary as a consequence. Naturally, the principles of treatment also differ (one method "supplementing qi and nourishing yin", the other method "resolving phlegm and removing dampness").

Cancer of lung, for example, can be classifies into such types as deficiency of both qi and yin (a morbid condition characterized by exhaustion of both yin fluids and yang, usually seen in the late stage of epidemic febrile disease and chronic consumptive diseases), and the type of phlegm-dampness. This is entitled as "treating the same disease with different methods" in Chinese medicine. In addition, for those patients suffering from different types of cancer, they were found to share the same "syndrome" in a certain stage of the illness (for example, the syndrome of insufficiency of the spleen-qi, hypo function of the spleen - a morbid condition chiefly manifested with decreased digestion and absorptive functions), Chinese medicine will apply the same treatment method of "strengthening the spleen and replenishing qi" to them. This is entitled as treating different diseases with the same therapeutic principle. Thereby, the whole body receives proper treatment.

(2).The combination of the method "strengthening the body resistance" with the method "eliminating pathogenic factors"

Whatever the employment of surgery, radiotherapy and anticancer agents, they all belong to the effective treatment against cancer (eliminating of pathogenic factors). However, due to their aim of destruction of cancer cells, in another word, their negative influence on the immunity of human body, they will inevitably bring about side effect, complication and sequel. In the design of the treatment scheme, it is necessary to take such factors into consideration as enhancing the comprehensive immunity of the patient himself / herself (namely strengthening the body resistance), repairing the injured cells and organizations to improve the resistance against cancer.

(3). Integral treatment VS. Partial treatment

For such cancers as skin cancer, nasopharyngeal cancer, and urinary bladder cancer, it is obliged to apply integral treatment. However, for terminal cancer with the proliferation of cancer cells to the entire body, the partial treatment enjoys priority in the treatment. Because of the poignant pain arising from the tuber compression, we should partially apply radioactive treatment to soothe the emergent symptoms of the patients.

During the course of partial treatment as operation and radioactive treatment, Chinese medicine can be employed for the repair and opsonic treatment of the entire body. Currently this perception of extending partial treatment to integral treatment turns out to be the most promising approach in many people's perspective.

Table 2 Comparison of the treatment effect between the respective employment of Tian Xian Liquid, radiation therapy and the combined application of chemotherapy and Tian Xian Liquid

(Comparison of treatment effect between combined employment of Tian Xian Liquid and the radiation therapy with the private radiation therapy)

Effect / Group	Number of cases (people)	Cure	With distinctive effect	Effective	Non-effective	Total of the effective
Combined	20	13(people)	6	1	0	20
		65%	30	5	0	100
Private	20	6(people)	6	8	0	20
		30%	30	40	0	100

(Comparison between [Tian Xian Liquid 1350ml + full dose DT6000cgy-7500cgy irradiation] and [private full dose of DT6000cgy-7500cgy irradiation]). (approximately P=0.01)

(Comparison of treatment effect between combined employment of Tian Xian Liquid and chemotherapy with the private chemotherapy)

Effect / Group	Number of cases (people)	Cure	With distinctive effect	Effective	Non-effective	Total of the effective
Combined	48	14(people)	12	12	10	38
		29.2%	25	25	20.8	79.2
Private	56	2(people)	22	8	24	32
		3.6%	39.2	14.3	42.9	57.2

Comparison between [Tian Xian Liquid + POD, PCD2 anticancer agents] and [private POD,PCD2 anticancer agents]

Cure:complete disappearance of tum or Distinctive effect: above 50% of tumor shrinkingEffective: 50% of tumor shrinking Non-effective:tumor development-- enlarge

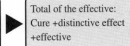

Total of the effective: Cure +distinctive effect +effective

(4). Comprehensive treatment

Only with the combination of medical treatment and the scientific management of entire life can the treatment of cancer remain fruitful. After surgery or in the course of receiving radiotherapy or anticancer agents, the patients should be in regular diet, live in a regular way with proper exercises to achieve a satisfactory therapeutic result and avoid recurrence. Therefore, an overall treatment should include the living-style management in the period of convalesence.

(5). Short-term treatment VS. Long-term treatment

In designing the project of long-term treatment, we should gradually apply the treatment in accordance to the state of development. In another word, adopting different approaches in different stages. The emphasis shall not lie on the short-term result, but on preserving and consolidating the therapeutic effect, on preventing from recurrence and transference, as well as on the recovery of long-term normal life.

42

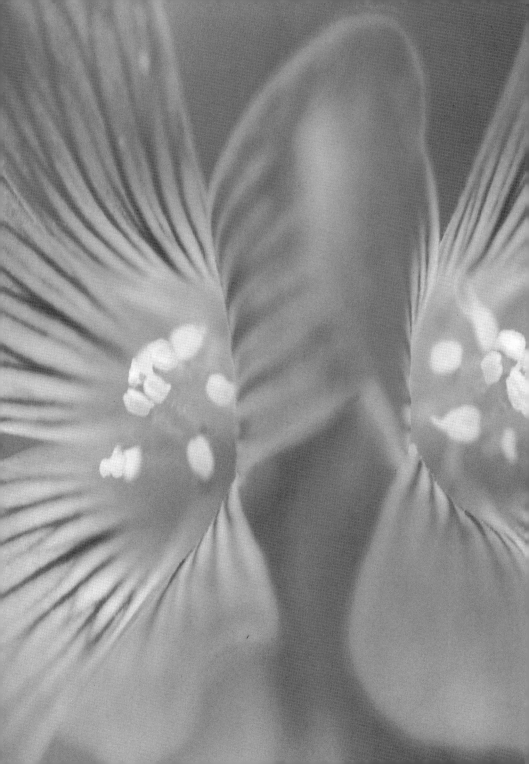

Chapter II

"Tian Xian Liquid"-Traditional Chinese Anticancer Medicine

45

Traditional Chinese Medicine rerecognized by the Chinese government

Although almost all of the traditional Chinese Anticancer Medicine entitles itself as "a secret

prescription handed down in the family from generation to generation", "peculiar prescription", the series of "Tian Xian" medicine such as Tian Xian Liquid or Tian Xian pill has undergone strict testing and research of pharmacological action. Plus its long-term clinical experiment in a large scale, it has been nationally recognized as the traditional Chinese anticancer medicine together with the approval from cancer patients.

Developing from the theories of Chinese medical and pharmaceutical theories, the series of Tian Xian medicine falls into the category of "complex han prescription ". Specifically speaking, the series of Tian Xian medicine abide by the theories of promoting the circulation of qi（a therapeutic method to relieve stagnation of qi by using medicines with the effect of regulating qi）; Promoting blood circulation by removing blood stasis (a method to treat blood stasis by using blood-activating and stasis-eliminating medicine); resolving the hard lumps, softening and resolving hard mass (a therapy for masses formed by accumulation of phlegm and blood stasis by using mass-

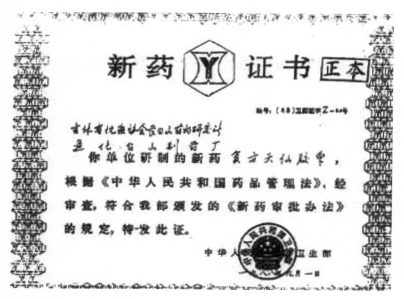

dissolving and blood-stasis-resolving medicine); clearing away heat and toxic material (a therapy for discharging heat and toxic qi accumulated in the body); eliminating dampness and removing the phlegm (a therapy to eliminate the pathogenic dampness and thick phlegm in the body); and removing the necrotic tissue and promoting granulation (a therapeutic method to removing the putrid tissues and promoting the growth of new tissues). The medicine pays special attention to the direct attack to cancer cells.

On the other hand, due to its direct attack against cancer cells as well as the effect of "eliminating pathogenic factors", Tian Xian medicine also provides such functions as strengthening the spleen and stomach (improving the function of protecting digestive system); tonifying the liver and reinforcing the kidney (supplementing the functions of the liver and kidney and nourishing the liver); invigorating qi and enriching the blood (a method to supplement the resource of body and reinforce hemotopoiesis); regulating yin and nourishing yang (a method to adjust the body balance), etc. In this way, the previous immunity of the body to cancer will be enhanced and thus the vital qi will be cultivated.

In the modulation of the series of Tian Xian medicine, the following theories of the traditional Chinese medicine are honored: channel tropism of property and flavor (property refers to such four properties as cold, heat, damp and cool; while flavor indicates hot, sweet, acid, bitter and salty; with its special drug effect, it acts in the special meridians and bowel), and the lifting, lowering, floating, and sinking (theory of direction of the action of drugs. The lifting and floating drugs with upward and outward effect are used for activating vitality, inducing sweating and dispelling cold. The lowering and sinking possess a downward and inward effect, and are used for tranquillizing, consolidating, or purgation), etc, as well as the principle of monarch, minister, assistant and guide (the different roles played by different ingredients of a prescription in their action. Monarch refers to principal drug, which produces the leading action to treat the cause and the main symptoms of a disease. Minister refers to adjuvant drug that helps strengthen the action of principal drug. Assistant refers to the adjuvant drug that helps offset side-effects and Conductant drug refers to the drug that directs the action of a prescription to the affected channel or tempers the action of other drugs).

Over 30 medicinal institutes and science institute around the world have conducted clinical observation over pharmacology, drug action, and toxicology of the series of Tian Xian Medicine. The series of these products are not only proved by scientific documents of its superior effectiveness, but

47

also the extensive application in respect of cancer treatment. In another word, among all the anti-cancer drugs developed across the world, the series of Tian Xian products enjoys the fame of traditional Chinese anticancer medicine with most favorable comments.

The development of Tian Xian Liquid

I was motivated to challenge "cancer" accidentally by my experience as an intern. I once saw a 12-year-old girl knelt down before a physician, crying heart-brokenly, "Doctor, please save my mother! Please!". At the end of my tether, I stood aside and helplessly saw the precious life of the girl's mother deprived by the terminal liver cancer. At that moment, I was determined to devote to fighting against cancer. I have full confidence on traditional Chinese medicine of its effect on curing the cancer.

I started my journey with collecting herbs and prescriptions "capable of treating cancer", as well as the folk treatment spreading from one generation to another around the country. Then I was engaged in the comprehensive research of anticancer drugs in a variety of aspects. During this period of time, I gathered nearly 1200 types of crude drugs and prescriptions according to the medical theories of Chinese medicine. In addition, all of the crude drugs and prescriptions are classified by the four theories of removing heat and toxic material; promoting blood circulation by removing blood stasis, alleviating pain and dissolving lumps, and invigorating qi and enriching blood.

The effect differs with different assortment and prescription of crude drugs. For example, assorting crude drugs A and B with opposite effects with the proportion of 1:1 or 1:3, or further plus C and D, no matter add or decrease one spoonful of this delicate combination, the effect will be utterly unmatchable. This effect is entitled "duel effect". The effect of single type of crude drug might be common, however, the combination of two, three or more, the superior effect will greatly impress you.

There remained 60 types of qualified crude drugs surviving from the strict selection and filtering of over 1200 types of crude drugs as well as prescriptions. Then 30 types survived from another round of strict selection of 60 types of crude drugs. Mainly composed of crude drugs with high anti-cancer effect, the 30 types have effect on enhancing intestine and stomach, promoting diuresis, nourishing and strengthening, as well as improving immunity. The function of each crude drug can be clearly defined.

Ultimately, over 18 years of thousands of hundreds of repeated combination and prescriptions of 30 types of crude drugs, we successfully found the Chinese anti-cancer medicine.

This research is fortunate enough to get the government's support and apply to the large-scale clinical experiments. In 1995, China National Ministry of Sanitation and National Science Committee, formally rated the initial product "Tian Xian Pill", which was spoke highly of by the Chinese government, as the key research projects of science and technology.

It is also approved to put into production as the new anticancer agents in the nation level. In 1998, it is ratified as Chinese medicine with satisfactory anti-cancer effect for the first time. On the basis of "Tian Xian Pill", we further developed the series of Tian Xian products of different systems, types and doses according to the medication course. Hopefully, we expect that this can effectively meet the requirements of all cancer patients.

Above all, the most important research subject lies on the liquefaction of Tian Xian pill. In 1991, the crude drugs through sustained research;

experiments and processing ultimately initiated the liquefaction of Chinese anticancer medicine, and marvelously improved previous medical effects. In order to stress the magnificent feat of "initiation", we named it as "China No. 1".

Therefore, from the "China No. 1 - Tian Xian Liquid", which is effective on a variety of cancers, to "China No. 1 - Tian Xian Liquid, refined type", up to the "China No. 1 - Tian Xian Liquid, strong type", which enjoys reinforced effect, we constantly strive for perfection in refinement and reinforcement. We hold it as our belief as well as mission of "persisting on research and development of more effective anticancer drugs to save the life of more cancer patients".

Main contents and constituents

the main crude drugs of Han prescription adopted by the series of Tian Xian products as Tian Xian Liquid and Tian Xian Pill derive from fresh herbs growing in the soil rich in trace elements. Therefore, they boast the effect of enhancing immunity system, among which such 14 herbs as ginseng, bighead atractylodes rhizome, and the root of large-flowered skullcap abundant in organic selenium and germanium that remain distinctively effective on the cancer of stomach, intestine and blood. Above all, the combination of several anticancer crude drugs enjoys most effective actions.

The Chang Bai Mountain -- "Treasure house of crude drugs"

All of the raw material of the series of Tian Xian products derived from the most precious herbs of the Mountain Range of Chang Bai. Please refer to

Table 3 Contents of main crude drugs of Tian Xian Liquid and respective actions .

Contents	Basicota and pharmacological actions
Ginseng	Basicota:refinement of the root of Five Jialse ginsengPharmacological actions:improvement of various body functions
Pearl	Basicota:refinement of the products of pearl oysterPharmacological actions:antianaphylaxis, stabilization, promotion of metabolism
Skullcap	Basicota: refinement of the root of fabaceceous skullcapPharmacological actions:dilation of blood vessel, lowering down blood pressure, enhancing immunity, diuresis, counter-poison, drainage, etc.
Black nightshade	Basicota:refinement of the leaves of black nightshadePharmacological actions:used as anti-cancer, anti-inflammatory, anti-virus and cordial agent,hypotensor
Bornel	Basicota: isolated from the resin obtained from Dipterpcarpaceae Pharmacological actions: acromatic stimulant for resuscitation and acceleration of blood stream. And can be used as an antipyretic and analgesic agent.
Bighead atractylodes rhizome	Basicota: dried root and stem of atractylodes,microcephala Pharmacological actions: used as hypoglycemic, antiseptic agent, anti-stasis of blood, anti-tumor. Promote diuresis and arrest spontaneous sweating.
Snakegourd root	Basicota: dried root of Trichosanthes kirilowii or cucurbi taceae.Pharmacological actions: used as anti-tumor and antiseptic agent
Clematis root	Basicota: dried root and rhizome of clematis chinensis, C. hexapetala or C. manshuricaPharmacological actions: relieve pain, used as antiseptic agent, prevent cancer in digesting organs.
Herba hedyotis diffusae	Basicota: dried root of hedyotis diffusaPharmacological actions: enhance immunity, anti-cancer actions. Promote accessory renal cortex.
Natural indigo	Basicota: drug consisting of a blue powder separated from the leaf of Baphicacanthus cusia. Indigofera suffruticosa, Polygonum tinctorium or Isatis indigotica.Pharmacological actions:used as anti-tumor and antiseptic agent, protect liver, promote digesting function of cells
Glossy privet fruit	Basicota: dried fruit of Ligustrum lucidumPharmacological actions: lowering lipogenesis of blood vessel, used as cordial, antitrussive and antiseptic agent, promote diuresis, enhance immunity
Licorice root	Basicota: dried root and rhizome of Glycyrrhiza uralensis, G. inflata or G. glabra Pharmacological actions: control immunity, relieve pain, used as an anti-trussive, anti-peptic ulcer, and anti-inflammatory agent
Dysuria	Basicota: dried sclerotium of porous plant DysuriaPharmacological actions: the avstracted material of Dysuria as well as polysaccharide of Dysuria can enhance immunity, and used as anti-tumor, diuresis and antiseptic agent
Zoogenetic bile	Basicota: refinement of zoogenetic bilePharmacological actions: relieve pain and used as an antiparasitic agent
Zoogenetic secretion	Basicota: dried secretion from the acromatic bladder of male animals. Pharmacological actions: increase blood stream of the heart, relieve pain, and used as antiseptic and anti-tumor agent.

51

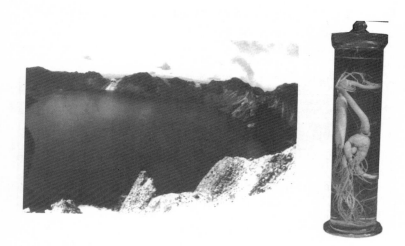

Table 3 for contents of main crude drugs and actions of Tian Xian Liquid.

Situated in the crater of the Mountain range of Chang Bai, the Chang Bai Mountain is an active volcano. Due to the constant eruption of the volcano, the extending mountain ranges are covered with thick volcanic ashes. Over years, the earth of the mountain range gradually accumulates over 20 trace elements such as selenium and germanium specially produced by the volcano. Other than indispensable constituents of the human body, these trace elements boast excellent effect on improving constitution, preventing from aging, latitude, and cancer.

In recent years, the dried Korean ginseng immersed in the natural fountain sprouting from the fault zone of the Chang Bai Mountian range has miraculously germinated. Besides, the residents near the Chang Bai Mountain enjoy longevity. It is said that this should be attributed to the fountain naturally sprouting from the Chang Bai Mountain Range.

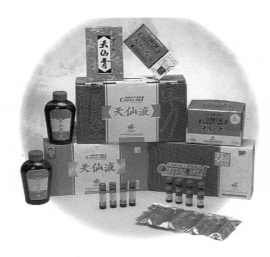

Therefore, the natural fountains of Chang Bai Mountain enjoy the fame of "every young mountain" in China. Due to the excellent nature of water, soil and climate of the mountain range, plants (herbs) in the neighborhood area grow rapidly with short growth cycle but long rest period. Then herbs with extraordinary characteristics are consequently cultivated.

Pharmaceutical actions of main crude drugs

(1). Ginseng

Outstanding effect on supplementing energy of the human body. In addition, the ginseng cultivated in the area abundant in water source plus soil of the Chang Bai Mountain Range contains at least 12 saponins, amino acid, polypeptide, polysaccharide, vitamin, and sodium, potassium, magnesium, steel, manganese, copper, zinc and germanium, etc.

In the animal experiment on researching the cancer pathogenic chemical material, we prove that with long-term consumption of ginseng, it can not only decrease occurrence rate of cancer, but also inhibit the growth of cancer cells. Besides, polysaccharide contained in ginseng can protect liver, improve immunity of the human body and reinforce the function of preventing from dissociation. With the combined employment of anticancer agents, other than improving therapeutic effect, it can also lessen the side-effects arising from the anticancer agents. It also boasts certain effect on the treatment of cancer of stomach and large intestine. According to the clinical experiments, the patients previously suffering from decline of white blood cell and of lymph corpuscles really achieved an increase of those after in-take.

(2). Skullcap

it contains polysaccharide, monosaccharide, flavone complex, mucolipid, trace elements, etc. According to recent medial research, skullcap was proved to be capable of improving comprehensive immunity and immunity against microbes of pathogeny, as well as reinforcing the actions of T lymph corpuscles. Polysaccharide can promote to induce interferon, enhance activation of esterification of T cells, improve the immunity of cells, as well as inhibit the growth of virus or cancer cells in the cell organization. As a result, most of it is used as an immunity-enhancing agent.

(3). Bighead atractylodes rhizome

Bighead atractylodes rhizome contains volatile oil and coumarin, etc.

According to the result of the experiment, the neutral oil of the volatile oil contained in the Bighead atractylodes rhizome definitely can inhibit the cancer of esophagus. And the volatile oil as a whole boasts an effect on inhibiting abdominal hydrops as well as on improving immunity. Due to its action of increasing white blood cell, it is mainly employed for preventing the side effects arising from the radiation and anti-cancer agents treatments in clinical experiments.

(4). Dysuria

Dysuria contains ergosterin, Polysaccharide, rough protein, inorganic salts and vitamin H, etc. among them, Polysaccharide is most effective as an anti-cancer agent mainly by reinforcing the polyphagia activation of macrophage. It is rare to separately use dysuria as an anti-cancer agent, but mainly for combined use with other agents of invigorating the spleen and removing dampness by diuresis in clinical experience. Therefore, it is usually applied to patients suffering form the cancer of retention of water. According to the clinical survey, with the combined use of anti-cancer agents, the condition of primary cancer of stomach can really be improved. In addition, it is proved that to be able to lessen the side effect of declination of immunity due to the use of anticancer agent. The separate employment of it or the extracted aim to improve the patients' immunity.

(5). Licorice root

Licorice root contains food sweating agent as well as the kalium and calcium salts, as well as flavones complex. According to the test result on animals, it is proved that polysaccharide of licorice root has effect on vesicular stomatitis virus, adenovirus III, herpes simplex virus I and vaccinia virus with distinctive inhibiting actions. Furthermore, according to the test result, glycyrrhizin acid as well as inducers can inhibit cancer of transplanted marrow as well as prevent the disease of white blood cell.

(6). Glossy privet fruit

Glossy privet fruit contains such elements as oleanolic acid, lupeol, mannitol, oleic acid, linolenic acid, palm oil and glyceride. Other than promoting the multiplication of lymphocyte in the basic experiment, it also can inhibit the declination of white blood cell arising from the radiation treatment and the use of anticancer agent. In the experiment of the cancer of cervices on the rats, the inhibiting rate of Glossy privet fruit reaches 49.2%.

(7). Natural indigo

Natural indigo contains indigo blue, etc, among which the effective anti-cancer ingredient is indirubin. Natural indigo can enhance the phagocytic function of mononuclear microphage of the animals suffering from cancer as well as the humoral immunity. In the respect of clinical experiment, it mainly emphasizes on the treatment and research of chronic leukemia, and consequently achieved distinctive therapeutic effect. With the combined use of anticancer agent and radiation treatment, the effect will be further enhanced, and naturally the side effect will be lessened.

(8). Radix trichosanthis

Radix trichosanthis contains starch, saponin, protein, and various amino acids. According to the test result of rats, it is proved that it has certain effect on abdominal hydrops of the liver cancer. Besides actions of lessening abdominal hydrops and extending longevity, it can also inhibit the transference of liver cancer. In clinic employment, it is mainly applied to treat malignant fetus monster and chorion cancer. The development and research of the series of Tian Xian products refers to the clinical employment against stomach cancer.

(9). Clematis root

Clematis root contains sterol, glucopipide, and saponin. Other than effectively inhibiting the tumor S180 in the experiment on rats, it can also be used to promoting blood circulation to remove obstruction in the channels, relieve pain, and eliminate dampness and phlegm. In clinical employment, it is mainly applied to the treatment of cancer of stomach, bones, and brain tumor.

(10). Black nightshade

Also entitled as Herba Solani Nigri. Such elements as black nightshade and saponin can effectively inhibit cancer of abdominal hydrops, lymphatic leukemia -615, as well as tumor 37, etc. in the clinical treatment; it is effective on the treatment of cancer of intestine, and lung.

(11). Borneol

Borneol possesses rather outstanding functions. Therefore, it can lead other drug constituent into the focus and relieve pain.

(12). Pearl powder

Pearl powder contains calcium carbonate, organic material as well as a variety of trace elements. With the employment of pearl power in the experiment on the yellow fruit fly as well as on rats, due to the respective declination of the lipofuscin of the heart and other organizations, it is proved to be effective on the removal of free radical (activated oxygen), and oxidized material.

(13). Herba hedyotis diffusae

Herba hedyotis diffusae contains cardiac glycoside, flavones, coumarin, etc. According to the test result, it has strong inhibiting effect on the cells of leukemia. During the course of immunity, rather than enhancing the resistance of the human body, the cancer focus would have no access to transference or nourishment. As a consequence, recurrence will be effectively prevented, which has a significant meaning on the treatment of cancer. Other than the distinctive enhancement of immunity, Herba hedyotis diffusae can further reinforce the phagocytosis of white blood cells and consequently enhance the immunity of body fluid. In addition, Herba hedyotis diffusae enjoys distinctive effect on inhibiting the cancer of cervix, the tumor S180 of the rats, lung cancer, cancer of abdominal cancer. Non-toxic.

(14). Secretion of the animal

Use Dried secretion of the animal as the agent. The pharmacological actions refer to the use as an antiseptic and anti tumor agent, increasing the blood stream of the heart, cardiac strength, and relieving pain.

There remains a long way for us to undertake of the treatment of cancer. Once stray form the correct direction, the life-long study will be negatively influenced. During the whole course of the treatment of cancer, the most vital element lies on the professional care provided by the medical groups, negotiations on the strategy of long-term treatment and recovery plan with joint effort as well as the gradual implementation of the plan.

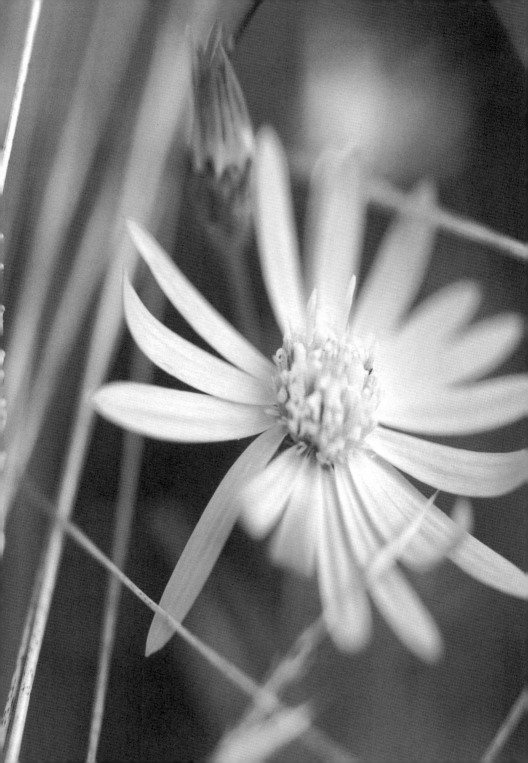

Chapter III

The effectiveness of treatments and precautions

63

From capsule to medicine liquid

Tianxian Pellet, the earliest progeny of Tianxian production, achieved the recognition "having the anticancer effects" of Tianjin Public Research Institute of Medicine Science. Later it was improved into the present "the Improved No.1 Tianxian Liquid in China". The course of study and development, which can be called the historic annual of Tianxian Liquid, shows as follows according to years.

In 1983, Tianxian Pellets were accomplished

In 1984, the clinicalal experiment result of Tianjin Research Institute of Medicine Science was published

In 1986, it was listed into the government development items of science and technology and put into planning

In 1986, Changbai Mountains Research Institute of Anticancer Medicine was set up in Tonghua, I was appointed director

In 1987, the Anticancer Association of Jilin Province and Changbai Mountains Medicine Research Institute were built up. I was appointed the director

In 1988, the clinical experiments of the State Cancer Center in USA affirmed that "the efficiency is over seventy percent"

In 1988, it was first authorized the treating medicine of cancer by Chinese government

In 1991, " No.1 Tianxian Liquid in China" was achieved

In 1995, "the Improved No.1 Tianxian liquid in China" was accomplished

In 1999, "the Enhanced The No.1 Tianxian Liquid in China" was put into study

In the topic of Tianxian Pellets research plan, the statement about the clinical experiments and pharmacological actions has achieved the ideal effects. The later research is the pharmacy, so I began to study the fluidization of Tianxian Pellets, which were filled into capsules at first.

It is well known that the things, which can make the intestines and stomach assimilate, digest fast and easily, should be, in the order of degrees, liquid for oral administration, capsule, troche. As a result, it is necessary to carry out the fluidization research.

In several clinical experiments of Tianxian Pellets, there is a problem that it is difficult for patients to take when they take the medicine because of different kinds of cancers, symptoms, etc.

For example, the patients whose physical abilities have exhausted have trouble in taking capsules. The apparatus of the patients in the final phase of cancer are too weak to take even a tiny one.

Furthermore, it is time-consuming for capsules to dissolve and also slow to be assimilated. The capsules may easily cause hydrochloric acid in gastric juice, sickness, vomiting, diarrhoea,etc.

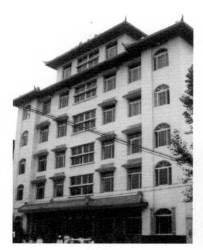

▲The Anticancer
Association in Jilin
Province

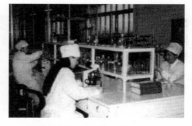

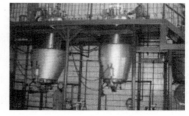

▲The factory of Changbai
Mountains Medicine
Research Institute

To Improve the Quality

The most direct way to solve problems is fluidization. The study will soon be carried out. In the meantime it is thought necessary to improve the effects of ingredients and coordination.

For an instance, the study of fluidization sprang to relearn the quality of new ingredients and the coordination effects, as well as to pay more attention to the subtle coordination rates. However, the ingredients are basically the same as those of Tianxian Pellets.

With regard to relearning the quality of new ingredients, the effects of the fresh herbs picked from Changbai Mountais are over one time better than the crude drugs made with the dry herbs, even the animal crude drugs, after the

We have sent Tianxian Liquid, which was made through three years' research, to more than thirty medical organs, university hospital in Beijing, Tianjin, Jilin, etc, so that they can carry out the clinical experiments. The diagram (IV) shows the medical effects in allusion to seven kinds of cancers' clinical experiments and six hundred and ninety-six cases, especially of the final esophagus cancer, stomach cancer and intestines cancer and so on. The result discovers that its effects are better than expected. Among them the effects to esophagus cancer, stomach cancer and intestines cancer are over ninety percent.

The Praises are Pouring in

According to the result of the clinical experiments, it is obvious that the Liquid enjoys high credits than the pellets. The praises are coming out everywhere. The exploitation of Tianxian Pellets and Tianxian Liquid at first

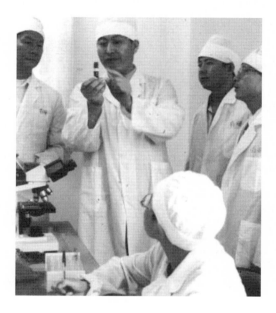

won the prize of the Best Products in Asian Pacific Region, and the Golden Prize of the second International Exposition held in Beijing. Then in the thirty-eighth World" Fair for Invention in Urika, they became the first Chinese to win the Highest Invention Prize for individual research.

After the exploitation of fluidization, the embolic agents "Tianxian Embolism" and plasters "Tianxian Plasters" are studied one by one. Tianxian Embolism can make the sufferers, who are growing weaker and weaker and unable to eat, to assimilate directly and easily. As to the stomach, esophagus, bronchus, thyroid gland and other apparatus near to the skin, all of which

Diagram (4) the medical effects to the final serious cancers

Name of Cancers	Number of Cases	Number of Effective	Persons Number of Ineffective Persons
Esophagus Cancer	225 (people)	201 (people)	24 (people)
Stomach Cancer	376	334	42
Intestines Cancer	95	85	10
Sum	696	620	76
Lung Cancer	94	73	21
Liver Cancer	34	25	9
Breast Cancer	78	56	22
Brain Cancer	46	28	18

The effect rate of the above diagram

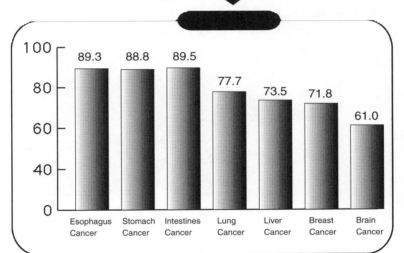

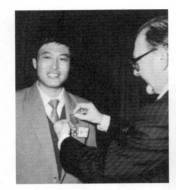

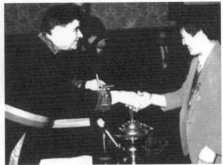

come with pains, the plasters are more suitable. Tianxian Plasters can effectively cure partially and alleviate pains, for Tianxian Plasters can penetrate the skin cells. No matter what kind of products will you choose, if you use it with Tianxian Liquid together, the effect will be doubled.

The above products are " Tianxian series of products". The following text will state the characteristics of each product.

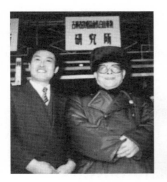

71

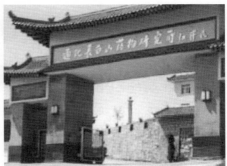

The Characteristics of the Improved of No.1 Tianxian liquid

The characteristics of The Improved of No.1 Tianxian liquid (called Tianxian Liquid in the following text), is based on the effects of " heat clearance, poison relief, blood moving, pain ceasing, spirit and blood nourishing" according to herbalist medicine. It aims to attack the bad genes and protect the good.

(I) The effect of killing cancer cells

The ingredients of Tianxian Liquid can control the growth of cancer cells, but also prevent the multiplication. Its effects mainly show in the following respects:

When the cancer cells begin its period multiplication, the Liquid will stop and kill it.

The Liquid can prevent their metabolic stages and make it distinguish.

The Sussus can destroy cellularities and make them to dissolve and disappear.

(II) The effect of metabolic intercession

Tianxian Liquid can change the metabolic stages of cancer cells. At the same time when it controls the multiplication, it can improve the metabolic actions of the affected body to resist the attack of cancer.

(III) The effect of improving immunity

The purpose of the Liquid is to afford a situation to strengthen immunity, and to accelerate actions of NK cells. The effect can be called specific and nonspecific immunity improvements. The Liquid can improve the function of T cells and also contains the crude drugs which can improve the function of B cells, including Rehmannia glutinosa, Ganoderma lucidum, eleutheroside, astragalus, ginseng, etc., all of which have the function of specific immunity improvement. In addition, the things, which penetrate the mononuclear phagocyte system to improve the immunity, include the crude drugs of pachman, polysaccharide, ginsenoside, Radix Trichosanthis, etc, all of which have the function of nonspecific immunity improvement.

(IV) The effect of trace elements

The trace elements can improve the body's function, cure the pathology, drive the genetic factors and prevent the division of cancer cells. For example, the organic Selenium of trace elements has the function of restraining the cancer genes. When it restrains the liver cancer, it prevents the mid-period cell to division period. What's more, the organic Germanium can abduct the secretory white cells' transmitters, interrupt its secretion, stimulate defensive system and restrain the spreading and growth of the cancer cells.

(V) The effect and function

The effects and functions of Tianxian Liquid:

It is the traditional Chinese medicine (the pure Chinese medicines) of anticancer with the remarkable medical effect. In addition, its excellent effects can improve all kinds of cancers reduce the side effects of western medicine. It can not only kill the cancer cell, but also improve the immunity, which avoids of destroying heart, kidney, liver, hematopoiesis and hardly does any harm to apparatus.

The medical effects can be improved if radiation and chemical treatment are used simultaneously. The side effects can also be reduced. The sufferers' physical power can be improved.

Foe those sufferers at the final phase, it can improve the final symptoms, reduce pains, prolong the life, strengthen the ability of coexisting with cancer and quality of life, QOL. It can prevent atrophic gastritis and benign tumors becoming malignant tumors.

The Characteristics of the More Effective of No.1 Tianxian Liquid

The More Effective of No.1 Tianxian Liquid (called the More Efficient of Tianxian Liquid in the following text) is based on the Improved of No.1 Tianxian Liquid and introduces in the latest medicine-making technology. It has become the more efficient traditional Chinese medicine. With the proof of the experiments in the BRI Research Institute of USA and the FRC Research Institute of Taiwan, the More Efficient of Tianxian Liquid can restrain the spreading of cancer cells, but kill the cells more directly.

The characteristic statement is as follows:

"Wall-breaking Theory" is the latest theory of killing cancer cells. That is to say it has the strong penetrating effect, accelerates the cells to wreck and dissolve so as to restrains tumors.

With the special combination, it can destroy the cell nucleus of cancer cells, kill and restrain cancer cells, to bring the effects into full play.

Its poison prevention effect is more obvious and its effective period is much longer to various kinds of the cells of tumor strains.

It was composed of the natural crude drugs and seldom has any side effects. At the same time, it can improve the immunity and make the cancer symptoms disappear.

After using the radiation and chemical treatments, the function of preventing the divisions of cancer cells is fully played and the side effects are reduced. If a few Tianxian Pellets are used, the efficiency to kill the cancer cells will be improved.

It is extensively suitable for all kinds of cancers. The effects will become greater, if Tianxain Embolisms are used simultaneously.

The Characteristics of the No.1 Tianxian Pellets

(I) The mechanical theory of Tianxian Pellets' effects

According to the clinical experiments of cancer restraining out of and in animal bodies, it is agreed unanimously that the No.1 Tianxian Pellets (called Tianxian pellets in the following text) has the function of killing and restraining many kinds of malignant tumors. At present , the mechanical theories of various kinds of anticancer medicines are carried out hotly. In the later part we will state them with some instances.

The function of D restraining NA (TOP Isomerases) TOP

There are two kinds of TOP isomerases, which adjust the DNA structure. They are TOP I and TOP II, the necessary ferments in the division and multiplication of cells. If one of them is restrained the division and multiplication are restrained, which equals that the cancer cells are restrained.

In the study of Tianxian Pellets effects for restraining DNA/TOP, Professor Li Dehua of Tianjin Medicine Science Research Institute proves that Tianxian Pellets can have the obvious effects in restraining DNA/TOP. T8and T9 of the Pellets have the remarkable effects in restraining DNA/TOP II, DNA/TOP I, the cut DNA and the DNA, which have become the compounded protein. In other word, the result of research shows that Tianxian Pellets have crucial lethal effectiveness.

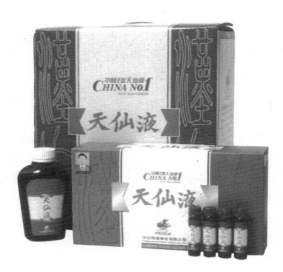

The active influence to DNA convergence and DNA model

Professor Wu and other people of the Basic Medicine Research Office in Guan Anmen Hospital of the Traditional Chinese Medicine Research Institute of China at first drew and made polymerase α from the ascitic fluid of a little mouse L1210. They then began to study Tianxian Pellets to it and discovered that Tianxian Pellets can obviously restrain polymerase α drew from the ascitic fluid of a little mouse L1210.

Basically, the degrees of restraining ferments of different tissues are generally same. As the medicine density is improved, the restraining rate is obviously increasing. All of this show that Tianxian Pellets have the strong restraining effects for DNA synthesis system

The influence to the period of cancer cells

Mr. Qu, etc, of the Tianjin Medicine Science Research Institute carried through the experiments and study of Tianxian Pellets' influence to the period of cancer cells. As a result, they found that to ascitic cancer cells and HeLa cells, the Pellets can increase the cells of period G2 and M and obviously reduce the cells of period G1 and S. Therefore it can be deduced that Tianxian Pellets can interdict the cell divisions of period G2 and M.

The function of improving the immunity

The countless clinical experiments prove that Tianxian Pellets can evidently improve the immunity system. As the Pellets build up the defensive function inside the body, they can bring the most effective results to restrain the cancer cells.

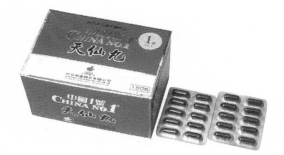

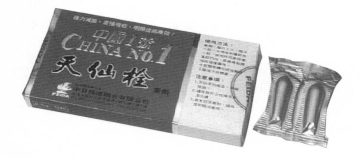

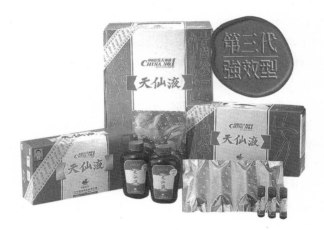

(II) The categories and different effects of Tainxian Pellets

In 1988, "the Compound Tianxian Capsules" (the present No.1 Tianxian Pellets of Tianxian series) achieved the affirmation of Chinese Government as being the traditional Chinese medicine.

The more effective prescriptions are invented with the continuous clinical experiments and combination of crude drugs. They are No.1, No. 3, No. 5, No. 6 and No. 7 Tianxian Pellets. The Charter V is for the reference of the characteristics of each one.

The characteristics of No.1 Tianxian Suppositorium of China

The biggest characteristic if that Tianxian Suppositorium can directly be absorbed by rectum mucosa, for the design of suppositorium. Tianxian Suppositorium passes through the rectum and does not pass through intestines and stomach, which can prevent gastric acid and other substances destroying the effective elements in the suppositorium to release the burden of liver. Usually, after thirty minutes' use, the suppositorium can filter into the blood and accelerate its circulation. The fast effect of the suppositorium has enjoyed the high praise. Furthermore, if the suppositorium is used with the fresh crude drugs, it can restrain the cancer cells and reduce the side effects of radiation and chemical treatment.

The main ingredients are alum, arisaema, dried toad, borneol, astragalus, sparganium, zedoary, hedyotis, secretio bufonis, camphol, which can detoxify, allay a fever, ease pain and disinfect and are suitable to treat esophagus cancer, stomach cancer, intestines cancer, lung cancer, liver cancer, Tzukung cancer, ovary cancer, prostate gland cancer, testis cancer, urinary cancer, breast cancer, vagina cancer, malignant lymph tumor and piles.

The characteristics of No.1 Tianxian Plaster in China

The main ingredients of No.1 Tianxian Plaster in China (called Tianxian Plaster in the following text) include arisaema, dried toad, bezoar, secretio bufonis, camphol, etc. Because the plaster can be plastered to the skin and the drug can be assimilated, its permeability is very strong. The plaster can control cancer cells and ease the stimulation of nerve and the pains caused by cancers.

81

Charter 5 the categories of Tianxian Pellets and main crude drugs and the effectiveness

	Ingredients	Effectiveness	Applicability
No.1 Tianxian Pellets	The root of Chinese trichosanthes, the seed of garden balsam. The dried venom of toads, black nightshade, trichosanthes root, clematis hedyotis, bezoar, umbellatepore funfus, etc.	To allay a fever, detoxify, soften and ease pain, nourish spirit and blood. To have the both effectiveness of radiation and chemical treatment	Esophagus cancer, stomach cancer, carcinoma of large intestine, gastro-intestinal cancer, etc.
No.3 Tianxian Pellets	Gineng, the tuber of dwarf lilyturf, jujube, the fruit of Chinese magnoliavine, astragalus, the dried rhizome of rehmannia, angelic, liquorice, etc.	To nourish spirit and blood, do good to spleen and stomach, alley a fever and detoxify, and to improve immunity	To ease side effects of radiation and chemical treatment, leukemia etc.
No.5 Tianxian Pellets	the bullb of fritillary, ginseng, lucid asparagus, the bark of official magnolia, cordate houttuynia, sun plant, the tuber of pinelli, liquorice, etc.	To benefit spirit, clear lung, reduce phlegm, clear stones, an to allay fever, ease pain relieve cough	Lung cancer, oral cancer, nasal cancer, throat cancer, brain tumor, etc.
No.6 Tianxian Pellets	Bezoar, capillary artemisia, Chinese thorowax, Ginseng, umbellatepore fungus, etc.	To allay fever, detoxify, reduce swelling, clear stones, open breath, stop pain	Liver cancer, gallbladder cancer, pancreas cancer, cirrhosis acute and chronic hepatitides, etc.
No.7 Tianxian Pellets	Centipede, whole worm, antler, apiary, ginseng, mountain arrowhead, selfheal, etc.	To nourish blood, clear stones, open breath, stop pain and improve benign tumors	Breast cancer, ovary cancer, Tzukung cancer, thyroid cancer, kidney cancer, bone cancer, prostate cancer, testis cancer, bladder cancer, penis cancer, skin cancer, etc.

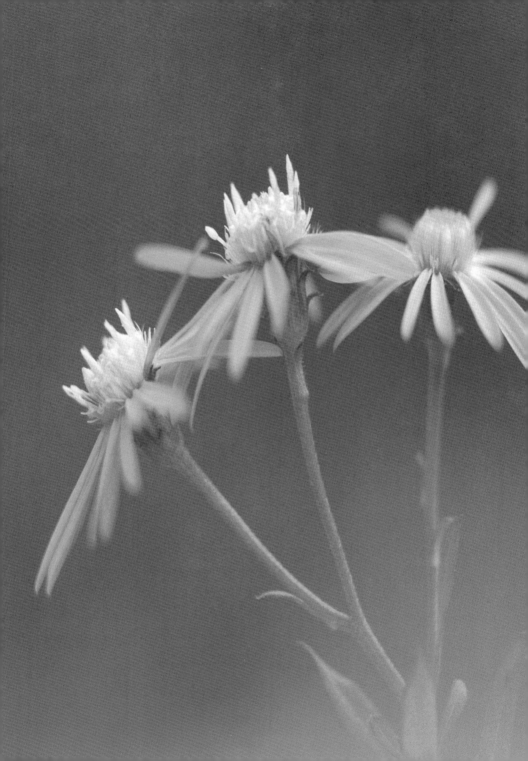

Chapter IV

The clinical experiments prove the effectiveness

The clinical experiments of ten research institutions

In this chapter, we will introduce the concrete clinical research and the dates and materials of experiments and probe into Tianxian Liquid and the effectiveness of its clinical treatment. Because the results have been written into the research thesis, it is still difficult to state them in the simple and easily-understood words. It does not matter for readers to skip this part, as long as readers know that any result of the clinical experiments can show the excellent anticancer effects.

From 1984 to 1996, the experiments were carried through in more than thirty cancer research institutions and special organs, such as American State Cancer Center, Chinese Medicine Research Institute of China, Tianjin Medicine Science Research Institute and so on. The experiments are about toxicology and pharmacy. All the study shows that the security and excellent anticancer effectiveness of Tianxian Liquid. Even though the patients take the Liquid chronically., it will not do any harm to the main internal organ apparatus, such as red blood cells, white blood cells, blood platelet, heart, liver, kidney, etc.

Charter 6 the main anticancer effectiveness and functions of Tianxian Liquids

(1)The barrier function to cancer cells

The ingredients of Tianxian Liquid erect barriers to the cancer cells and make them unable to continue multiplication, at the growing phase of cancer cells1.

1. It can stop cancer cells multiplying and make them die at some time of the multiplication period.

2. It can impede and stop the breathing function of cancer cells, then the cells will die at some time of the cells' energy metabolism.

3.It can destroy cancer cells and make them dissolve and die.

(2)The function of adjusting metabolism

The liquid restrains the multiplication of cancer cells by changing the various kinds of metabolisms, which are necessary for the multiplication of cells. Inthe meantime, it can improve the metabolisms of the organisms affected by cancer cells and their anticancer ability. Correspondingly, the multiplicatio of cancer cells the crude drugs owning the function of adjusting metabolism black nightshade, climbing nightshade / angelica, the root of red-rooted salvia.

(3)The function of great immunity improvement

The liquid can adjust the internal conditions so as to make the immunity function, which is improved as the multiplication of cancer cells is restrained come into being easily. In result the acting ability of cell killers. the crude drugs owning the function ginseng, pachman, Chinese honey locust, the root of Chinese trichosanthes, etc.

(4) The functions of trace elements   The movements of trace elements can change the organism's physiology and drive the genetic cells to move to destroy the cancer cells.

1. Se: the genetic cells of organic Se have the restraining function, control cancer cells and then prevent the mid-period cells beginning to divide

2. Ge: Ge can accelerate the secretions of the soluble substance II of lymph and interferon I, stimulate the autoecious anticancer function and control the growth and pervasion of tumors

The anticancer medicine with extensive usages

Tianbxian Liquid has the apparent restraining function and affect the DNA compounding period of cancer cells. It is certain that its restraining rate can reach 40% to 89.1%. As for the clinical experiments for the sufferers, who have not received operation, the radiation and chemical treatments, and 696 patients, who are suffering the telophase esophagus cancer and stomach cancer and have recurred after treatments, it is found that the liquid can restrain the growth of cancer cells, after they took Tianxian Liquid. The concrete dates include 2.6% complete relief (tumors disappear completely), 9.3% partial relief (tumors decrease more than a half) and 77.2% stability (tumors decrease less than a half and cancer cells do not increase).

What's more, Tianxian Liquid has the excellent effectiveness to improve the patients' condition and has greatly solved the anorexia problem of esophagus cancer sufferers and symptoms of pain, and so on. To the esophagus cancer suffers, Tianxian Liquid, radiation treatment (725 cases) and the chemical treatment (131 cases) are used together in the clinical experiments, double effects are achieved that the complete relief of radiation treatment increases by 28.3% (P<0.1) and that of the chemical treatment increases by 25% (P< 0.05). Therefore, it is certain that Tianxian Liquid can improve the effectiveness of radiation and chemical treatments.

In addition, in the study of immunity pathology, if the esophagus cancer sufferers take Tianxian Liquid before the operation, it is found that the reaction of the cells inside and outside lymph and phagocytes will become strong after the tumor samples cut in the operation are studied through pathologic histology and electron microscope, while the cancer karyons and its cells begin to degenerate and the necrosis appears.

According to the above clinical experiments, it is can be said that Tianxian Liquid is a kind of medicine with extensive usages, especially the separated treatment to the telophase cancers, it can be used with the chemical treatment and radiation treatment and the ideal Chinese medicine to prevent cancer recurring and transferring.

(I) The experiments of animal toxicology
Little white mouse

If the little white mouse takes Tianxian Liquid, the absolute lethal dose is 18.2G/kg, the smallest lethal dose is 9.1g/kg and there is no obvious slow toxicity. In addition, LD50 (the short name for Lethal Dose, meaning a half of lethal dose) is 13.62 ± 1.6g/kg (charter VII). The lethal reason is the breathing difficulties.

Big white mouse

Experiment (I) of big white mouse

First, the big white mice are respectively fed on 3.5g/kg, 2.8g/kg, 22.6g/kg, 18.4g/kg, 15.3g/kg of Tianxian Liquid. After a week's observation, the obvious toxic reaction is not found.

Experiment (II) of big white mouse

Each mouse is fed on 4.21g/kg.every day. The total time is ninety days. The weights of the big mice of the medicine-using group are growing more slowly than those of the non-medicine-using group and there is no obvious influence to the functions of red blood cells, white blood cells, blood platelet, heart, kidney, liver, etc. With the biological dissections and contraction of the

Charter VII Parameter of the acute toxic experiments of Tianxian Liquid to little white mice

The absolute lethal dose	18.2(g/kg)
The minimal lethal dose	9.1(g/kg)
The shortest time to die after taking	4 hours
The longest time to die after taking	3 days
The average surviving time of dead animals	15 days
The time for toxic animals to become natural	15 days
LD50	13.62 ± 1.6(g/kg)

(*notes) the experiment group of Kunming mice arranges 7 phases of dispensing dose and investigate the conditions of 10 mice. The maximal dose is the maximal dose. The dose reduces by 0P×1 at 1:07. the group observes the weight for 6 days after the medicine has been taken for 3 days, then calculate LD50 with Probity unit (average 5, having the normal variable with standard warp 1)

mice of forty-five days and those of ninety days, there is no apparent damage.

Cat

The cats respectively take 0.7g/kg, 0.6g/kg of Tianxian Liquid. More than half of the two groups of cats vomit in several hours after taking the medicine. At the same time, there are changes on the electrocardiograms and the movements of their hearts become slow. The hearts of 1/3 of the excessive medicine-using group are damaged by the conduction Block III. The symptoms of ventricular reaction appear, such as digitalis (used as cardiac stimulant, the medicinal plant originating from Europe). Then the cats die. The surviving cats turn to be natural in seven hours after they are fed on Tianxian Liquid. According to the above acute toxic reaction, Tianxian Liquid belongs to the medicine without toxicity in principle. The hypersensitivities to toxic reactions of various kinds of animals are different. In addition, the patients who take the digitalis cannot take this medicine.

(II) The function of cell toxicity

Tianxian Liquid is made from the crude drugs with the strong toxicity (the root of Chinese trichosanthes, indigo, hedyotis, blacknightshade, etc). The experiments of American State Cancer Center prove that Tianxian Liquid has the cell toxicity to ten kinds of cancers (lung cancer, breast cancer, leukemia, Zhivay mother cell tumor, kidney cancer, malignant melanoma, brain cancer, stomach cancer) and forty-eight kinds of cancer cell strains. It can not only stop the protein compounding, which is necessary for the growth of cancer cells, but also impede the multiplication period of cancer cells. Further it accelerates cancer cells to dissolve and distinguish. The lethal ability of Tianxian Liquid to cancer cells has relation with the density and the term of validity.

(III) The influence to the cell period and DNA compounding

The characteristic of Tianxian Liquid' effectiveness to cancer tumors is that it can directly affect the DNA compounding of cancer tumor cells. On the basis of density differences, Tianxian Liquid can restrain the DNA compounding of HeLa cells (a kind of cancer cells, found in a Tzukung cancer sufferer by Doctor Gorge Gale of John Hopkins Hospital in 1951), but change the multiplication period of cancer cells. As Charter 8 shows, the liquid with the density of 10~20mg/ml, it can prevent the divisions of the cells in the period G2 and M, and most of HeLa cells appears to be in the period of G2

Charter 8 The influence of Tianxian liquid to HeLa cells and DNA contents

Cell period	G1(%)	S (%)	G2, M (%0
Object group	25	60	15
Tianxian Liquid 10 μ g/ml	6	50	44
20 μ g/ml	1	19	80
30 μ g/ml	17	60	23
40 μ g/ml	78	20	2

and M. if the density increases to 40mg/ml, it can obviously restrain the DNA compounding of cancer cells and even the DNA of cancer cells will decrease. The cells of the period G1 and M are hypersensitive to radiations. Tianxian liquid has the obvious effects of restraining and lethal ability to cancer cells of the period G2 or M, if it is used with radiation treatments. Tianxian Liquid shows the obvious restraining function to DNA/TOP of human body. The forming of the marker with these ferments can restrain the compounding of protein. In other word, it will destroy DNA.

(IV) The strengthening effectiveness to radiation treatment

We use the anoxia HeLa cells and the forming way of performing colony (a kind of segregated thallus or the multiplied cell colony in the growth mediums) to study the effectiveness to radiation treatment. With the counting of Seven Coulombs (to take the charge S1 as an unit, the charges transferred in one minute by current A1 added the fixed number equals the charges of 18 times of 6.25 *10) and the computer simulation, the typical way of attacking markers once. The life curve of cells treated with A, B equation indicates that Tianxian Liquid has the strengthening effectiveness. However, when Tianxian Liquid improves the effectiveness of radiation treatment, if must be based on radiation amount.

(V) The restraining function to the testing tumors

The experiment is carried out, in which mice and weasels are transplanted with the adrenalin entity of tumor S180, adrenalin ascites carcinoma, ruminant stomach (the first stomach of ruminant), flat tumor, lung cancer Levis, mouse leukemia L1210. Thirty days later, the cancer tumor planted group is divided into two, one is Tianxian Liquid group and the other is the non Tianxian Liquid group (the average diameter of cancer tumors in the non Tianxian Liquid group is 8.1mmt, while the average diameter of cancer tumor in Tianxian liquid group is 8.6mm). the dose of Tianxian Liquid group is 2-5g/kg once every day and the total time is twenty-one days. Twenty-four hours later counted from the last doe, the animals of each group begin to die and then the weight of tumors. The result show that the restraining rates of Tainxian Liquid to solid tumor and flat proventriculus tumor are 58.7 (P<0.01) to 2g/kg and 89.1% (P<0.001) to 5g/kg (Charter IX).

(VI) The dates of the clinical cases in the cancer treatment

In the clinical experiments, the sufferers of the telophase peptic cancer are continuingly given the medicine. 10 ml of the medicine is given three times a day.

Charter 9 The effectiveness of Tianxian Liquid to cancer in the common mice experiments

Kinds of tumors	Number of mice	Dose(g/kg)	Oral dose	Restraining rate and surviving days
S180	¡@¡@¡@¡@¡@¡@10	2	21	35.6%
	10	5	21	48.3%
	10	Comparing groups	21	–
Adrenalin entity	9	2	18	54.9%
	9	5	18	57.6%
	9	Comparing groups	18	–
Lung cancer Lewis	5	2	20	46.9%
	5	5	20	56.4%
	5	Comparing groups	20	–
flat proventriculus tumor	6	2	21	58.7%
	6	5	21	89.1%
	6	Comparing groups	21	–
adrenalin ascites carcinoma	10	2	18	8.0days
	10	5	18	7.5 days
	10	Comparing groups	18	–
L1210	6	2	14	8.2 days
	6	5	14	8.4 days
	8		14	–

93

Charter 10 The effectiveness of single use of Tianxian Liquid for telophase cancers

Names of tumors	Number of cases	The effective (case)	The useless (case)	Effectiveness rate
Esophagus cancer	225	201	24	89.3
Stomach cancer	376	334	42	88.8
Intestines cancer	95	85	10	89.5
Lung cancer	94	73	21	77.7
Liver cancer	34	25	9	73.5
Adenoma of breast	78	56	22	71.8
Brain tumor	46	28	18	61.0

(VII) The dates the clinical experiments of single use of Tianxian Liquid for peptic carcinoma

More than thirty medical organs in Beijing, Tianjin, Shanghai carry through the clinical experiments of Tianxian Liquid to 696 cases of telophase esophagus cancer, stomach cancer, intestines cancer. The evaluation assures that the effective cases are 620 except the cancers of stable period according to the present standard of China. It is also certain that Tianxian Liquid enjoys high effectiveness (charter 10)

(VIII) The clinical treatment to esophagus cancer with simultaneous uses of Tianxian Liquid and operation

If the patient of esophagus cancer takes Tianxian Liquid before operation,

Charter 11 the effectiveness rate of "900ml of Tianxian Liquid + half of DT4000cgy irradiation" and "single radiation with half of DT4000cgy irradiation"

Therapy Total	effectiveness rate (%)
Tianxian Liquid and Radiation	80
Single radiation	45

Charter 12 the effectiveness rate of " 1350ml of Tianxian Liquid + half of DT4000cgy irradiation" and "single radiation with half of DT6000~7500cgy irradiation"

Therapy Total	effectiveness rate (%)
Tianxian Liquid and Radiation	80
Single radiation	60

Charter 13 the effectiveness rate of "1350ml of Tianxian Liquid + half of DT6000~7500cgy irradiation" and "single radiation with total DT6000~7500cgy irradiation"

Therapy Total	effectiveness rate (%)
Tianxian Liquid and Radiation	95
Single radiation	60

Charter 14 the effectiveness rate of "1350ml of Tianxian Liquid + total DT6000~7500cgy irradiation" and "single radiation with total DT4000cgy irradiation" to the esophagus cancers of middle and telophase.

Therapy Total	effectiveness rate (%)
Tianxian Liquid and Radiation	71.4
Single radiation	11.9

Charter 15 the contrast of the effectiveness of Tianxian Liquid + chemical anticancer medicament and single anticancer medicament to esophagus cancer

Therapy Total	effectiveness rate (%)
Tianxian Liquid + chemical anticancer medicament	79.2
Single anticancer medicament	11.9

Chapter 16 The rate of side effect caused by radiation therapy has been reduced by Tianxian Liquid.

Symptoms	Sickness and vomiting	Hair loosing	Catarrh	Reduction of white blood cells	Reduction of blood platelets	Reduction of hemoglobin
(%)	82.3	79.3	83.6	93.7	98.1	88.5

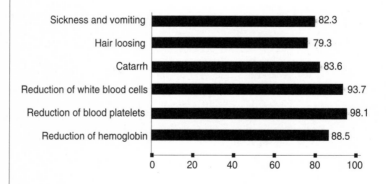

it is found that a great number of lymph cells have perked into the cancer tissues or the surrounding area of the cancer cells and the cancel cells begin to become necrotic after the samples removed in the operation are observed. At the same time, the karyons of cancer cells and the material cells start to degenerate. In result, it is sure that Tianxian can obviously improve the immunity. What's more, in some operation cases, the tissues around tumor become malacic and easy to fall off, which can make operation go along smoothly. Because Tianxian Liquid can greatly improve the immunity, the recurring rate after operation has decreased by 44% from 69% to 25% to removal operation and the cases of the residual and transfer tumor tissues.

(IX) The clinical treatment of the simultaneous uses of Tianxian Liquid and radiation therapy

The clinical treatments to the sufferers of esophagus cancers of middle phase and telophase with radiation therapies of different radioactive rays and Tianxian Liquid have been carried through. It can be deduced that the effectiveness has been greatly improved when the Liquid is used simultaneously according to the clinical dates. That is to say that Tianxian Liquid has the excellent restraining function to esophagus cancer (charter XI and XIV).

(X) The clinical treatment of the simultaneous uses of Tianxian Liquid and anticancer medicament

The experiment group and comparing group are arranged. Tianxian Liquid and anticancer medicament are used simultaneously to the sufferers of esophagus cancers of middle phase and telophase. The result shows that Tianxian Liquid can the short-period effectiveness of anticancer and the cure rate of esophagus cancer and also can restrain the side effects of arrest of bone marrow, etc caused by anticancer medicament (charter XV and XVI). In addition, the most attractive aspect is that lung cancer and lymphoma are eased in a short period after the Liquid is used together. The cure effectiveness of long -time is being studied in the clinical experiments. This item of experiment indicates that the simultaneous uses of Tianxian Liquid and chemical anticancer medicament can improve the cure rate of esophagus cancer to 25%.

(XI) the side effects of Tianxian Liquid

20ml of Tianxian Liquid is used once to the clinical exoeriments. Though 3% of patients feel uncomfortable with their stomachs and have a jaded appetite, the general come back and become natural and can take the Liquid continuingly. Furthermore, among the sufferers who take Tianxian Liquid only, there is no harm to their internal organs or apparatuses, such as liver, kidney, heart, lung, hematopoietic system, etc.

The living examples with various functions

The above dates come from the clinical experiments of American State Cancer Center, the Traditional Chinese Medicine Research Institute of China, Tianjin Medicine Science Research Institute, etc. Its result can be certified furhther. The ingredients of Tianxian Liquid have various kinds of functions, of the mechanical function about how to give play to the effectiveness becomes more obvious with these experiments.

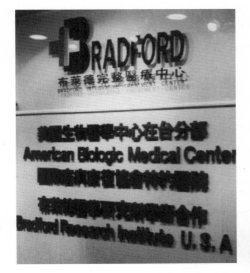

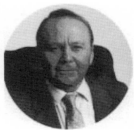

▲Doctor Blade Fort, the
director of BRI
Consortium Research
Institute of USA

For example, as for the mechanical function of crude drugs to cell toxicants, crude drugs can prevent the compounding of protein which is necessary for the growth of cancer cells, because they can confuse its multiplication period by directly affecting the compounding of DNA so that the dead cell membranes to dissolve by themselves.

On the other hand, the side effects are clearly reduced and the killing rate is also improved, when the radiation therapy and the Liquid are used simultaneously. Therefore, it is certain that the Liquid has the function to improve the sensitivity of radiation and to strengthen the lethal ability of radioactive rays.

The function to strengthen the effectiveness of white blood cells and various immunities is actually proved. The reason for the body activity is that "the purpose to increase hemoglobin is to improve the oxygen-supplying ability of red blood cells and to renew the vigor of blood". In other word, Tianxian Liquid can reduce the activity of free radicals (active oxygen). About the respect of the function of antioxidation, we can see the course of reducing the number of free radicals and peroxide lipin in patients' bodies.

In addition, Tianxian Liquid can actually restrain the activating of cancer cells, although we don not know what kind of ingredient it is and how to function to caner cells.

According to the above clinical experiments, Doctor Blade Fort, the pioneer and pundit in the field of free radical research all over the world and the director of BRI Consortium Research Institute of USA, brings forward the following statement and comes to a conclusion with the policy to use Tianxian Liquid in the clinical cases.

"Firstly, I suggest to perform operation or to use Tianxian Liquid when undergoing the anticancer medicament and radiation therapy. That is the basic policy o treat patients in my hospital. Of course, the safest way is to remove cancer cells. Though the anticancer medicament and radiation therapy have their specified effectiveness, they can not succeed in removing the free radicals. Sometimes they may accelerate their makings. In this respect, the function of antioxidation of Tianxian Liquid is most attractive. Moreover, Tianxian Liquid can improve the immunity and restrain the activity of cancer cells. There is no more ideal medicine than TianXian Liquid.

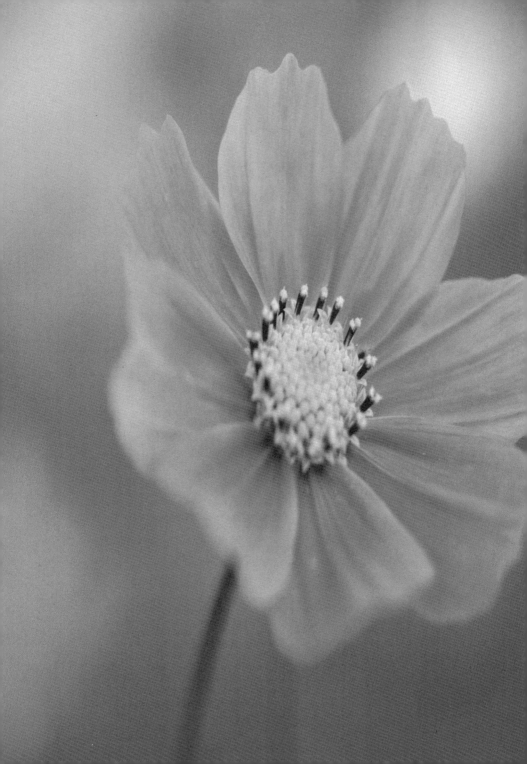

Chapter V

How to Prevent Cancer and Cancer Transfer

Re-adjust Daily Habit

For diseases such as cancer, treatment process can be accomplished successfully, while it cannot be cured thoroughly; also the possibilities for the disease to re-occur and transfer still exist. So the importance of routine health examination can be fully understood. Besides hospital examination, the self-observation of patients is also important.

Patients should pay attention to such signs in the original pathologic part as tumour, nodes, pains or not, whether anorexia, tired, losing weight, anemia, etc. Patients should report to doctor immediately when such abnormal phenomenon occur.

To re-adjust daily habit is more important for patients . The cause for cancer is various, it can be associated with such factors as daily accommodation, work, spiritual pressures, etc. just like Routine Diseases as diabetes and high blood pressure. So patients may re-adjust their daily habits and improve their living schedule as well:

Is your diet balance or not?

Drinking too much alcohol liquor?

Do you smoke?

Is your life style regular?

Are you disturbed by pressure?

Pay more attention to your health when such phenomenon happens.

Take foods that can prevent cancer

When you are considering to change your routine life style, daily diet is a very important aspect. various food contains materials that will cause cancer (includes pickle food, fumigated food and deep-fry food, etc.). Also there are various foods that have anti-cancer effects. So taking foods that can prevent cancer is beneficial and is necessary for cancer preventing. Forming such habits is important for improving diet structure.

Foods that can prevent cancer include

Melon and Fruits

Watermelon, Cushaw, Chinese watermelon, Balsam pear, Pawpaw, Apple, Pear, Lemon, Loquat, Mandarin orange, Tangerine, Orange, Banana, Grape, Fig, Haw, Ebony, Olive, Strawberry, Jujube, Walnut, Apricot, Peach, Mulberry

Vegetables and Seaweed

Garlic, Garlic bud, Shallot, Ginger, Sword bean, Cabbage, Bamboo shoot, Aubergine, Aubergine, Radish, Carrot, Bean sprout, Sea tangle, Sea tangle sprout, Sea moss, Pearl moss, Cress, Spinach, Celery, Tomato

Edible Mushroom

Agaric, Mushroom, Fungus

Cereal

Mung bean, Soybean, Wheat, Buckwheat, Corn, Cornmeal, Job's tears, Broomcorn

Animal

Loach, Sea cucumber, Crucian, Qinghua fish, Oyster, Clam, Field snail

Others

Honey, Sunflower seed, Bean curd, Buttermilk, Vinegar, Chrysanthemum, Tea

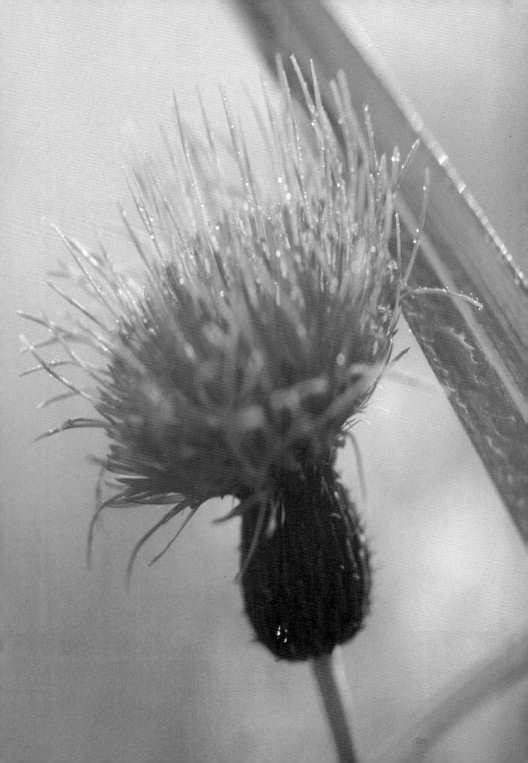

Appendix

Introduce to International Cancer Rehabilitation Association

An organization that support worldwide cancer-fighting patients

International Cancer Rehabilitation Association (Headquarter in Hongkong) is an organization that support worldwide cancer-fighting patients. As a representative of this organization as well as medical research member of China National Ministry of Health, I dedicate myself to the promotion of the association's global activities. Under assistance of Sino-japan Feida United Co., Ltd., we are taking varieties of activities with focus in headquarter Hongkong.

Now there are over 40 million people in the world who are suffering the pains brought by cancer. For the purpose of eradiating cancer in this world, International Cancer Rehabilitation Association are taking varieties of activities to achieve it's goal. In the area of south-east Asia where the medical condition is poor, we are disseminating relative knowledge of cancer, treatment solution and latest technology and therapeutics of cancer, also we are promoting activities concerning ways for preventing cancer.

In addition, the promotion activities and support for those people who are fighting with cancer is ongoing worldwide through cancer-related international conferences. In Japan, more than ten lecture and exercise meetings have been already taken.

Through activities and efforts by International Cancer Rehabilitation Association, "No Cancer" movement has been promulgated to the whole world. The efforts and various of activities will continue in the future.

Now I have the honor to introduce main branch institution of International Cancer Rehabilitation Association in the world.

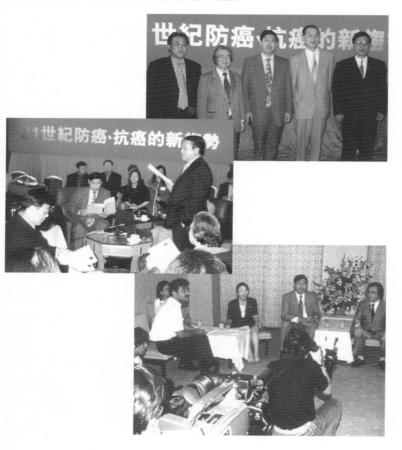

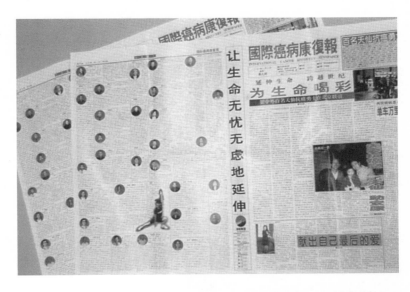

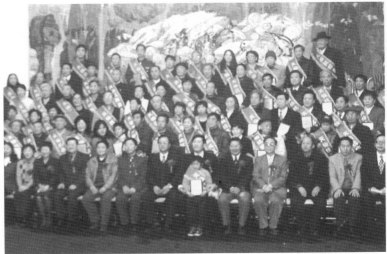

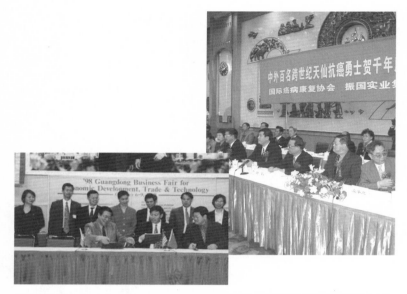

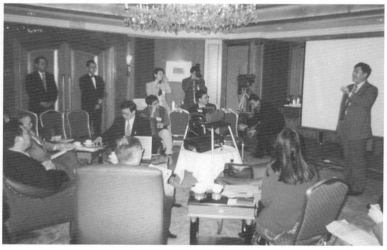

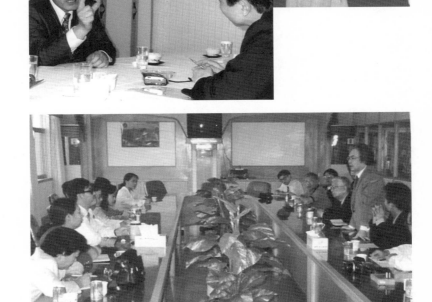

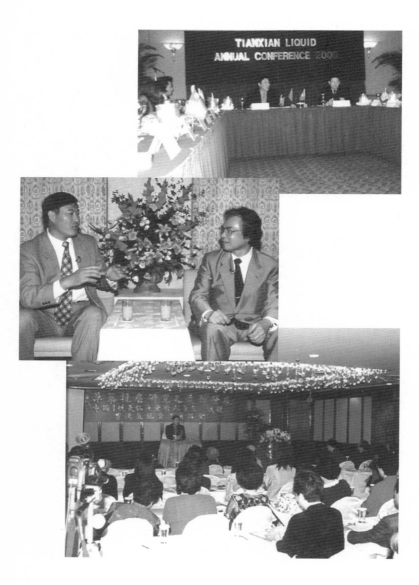

Contact Information on headquarter and branches of International Cancer Rehabilitation Association

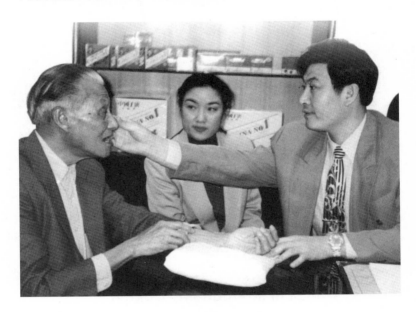

Headquarter of International Cancer Rehabilitation Association (Hong Kong)

8/F. HENCHY TOWER 9

CHATHAM ROAD T.S.T, KLN., HONG KONG.

TEL: (852) 2721 1555

FAX: (852) 2721 1000

Japanese Language Service: (852) 2368-1943

Homepage Address:

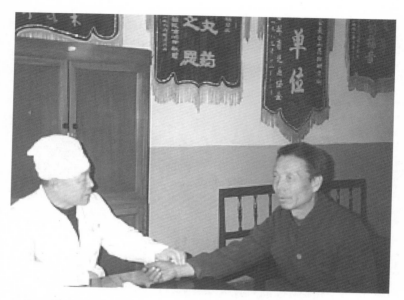

http://www.cjfeida.com

e-mail: lifecjf@cjfeida.com

Taiwan Branch of International Cancer Rehabilitation Association

TEL: (0080) 855 576

(Toll free from Taiwan to Hongkong, please dial directly, no need to add area code.)

Malaysia Branch of International Cancer Rehabilitation Association

TEL: (60) 3292 6682

Thailand Branch of International Cancer Rehabilitation Association

TEL: (66) 2264 2218

Philippine Branch of International Cancer Rehabilitation Association

TEL: (63) 2415 8714

US Branch of International Cancer Rehabilitation Association

Toll Free Call: (1) 800 810 0055

Japan Branch of International Cancer Rehabilitation Association

Wang Zhenguo Office, Japan

TEL: 03-5210 2246

FAX: 03 5210 4999

Homepage Address: http://www.tensen.com

Well-known Anti-cancer Effect of Tianxian Liquid

The research of Dr. R.W. Britford, director of US BRI Corp. Research Institute, has been described in Chapter Four of Section I, Dr. Britford is a pioneer as well as authority in the field of Free Radical (active oxygen) research. He believes that the cause of diseases originates from Free Radical. Through the analysis of Free Radical's amount and micrography of blood, various of diseases can be diagnosed. The theory and technique of this way is very complicated and professional, so I will not explain it in detail here. To be briefly, to calculate the amount of Free Radical in special method, and diagnose the health status or disease of patients, then observe the blood with special blood micrograph approach, so that the situation of diseases can be grasped.

Recently, people began to pay more attention to Free Radical, because Free Radical is considered to be the cause of cancer and other kinds of diseases. Now I would like to explain Free Radical to readers, when air comes into our body, oxygen will be transformed in our body through energy transition process, Free Radical is so called oxygenation-form oxygen. In ordinary condition, when virus invade human's body, the oxygenation materials will kill the invaded virus and bacteria. Free Radical will act as the role of Guard in our body.

Then why active oxygen is the cause of diseases? The problem is that there are too much active oxygen than normal standard. Promoting and evocative effects are two causes of cancer, while Free Radical contains both aspects concerning pathology factors. If Free Radical combines unsaturated fatty acid, it will be prime criminal for various chronic diseases and it will produce peroxid materials.

Dr. Britford and the Research Team began to measure the number of Free Radical, with reference of daily diagnoses and treatment, drew a conclusion that Free Radical is main cause for cancer as well as reason for worsen. When they are finding solution for eliminating peroxid materials, Chinese Herbal Medicine arise to their views and Tianxian Liquid was obtained.

From the beginning of eliminating peroxid materials and Free Radical, to concentration on Chinese Herbal Medicine, then Chinese Medicine, Finally Tianxian Liquid. Maybe most of research members are Chinese, Dr. Britford began to pay more attention to Chinese Medicine.

Then many procedures and various of tests have been taken. The elimination effect of Tianxian Liquid for Free Radical and peroxid materials has been proved, also anti-oxygenation function of Tianxian Liquid concerning anti-cancer effects is tested with the center of Dr. Britford as well as various of research by international research institutions.

The co-research project is taken by doctors of Chinese Tumour Society, professors of Bio-physics Research Institute, China Science Academy, Bio-chemical clinical PhD of Cliffland University, USA, as well as staffs of General Health Dep. Of Capital University, USA. After two years' research, the research paper was published both in Chinese and English. The paper is outlined in details and contains numbers of materials and data, it's an important and invaluable research fruits for us, the structure of the paper can be outlined as follows:

1.Experiment on eliminating Free Radical
Tianxian Liquid can eliminate various of Free Radical effectively.

Eliminate hyper-oxygen Free Radical, over 0.3 million SDD/ 1 cc

Eliminate Free Radical produced by leucocyte that Vitamin E has no effect on.

Eliminate Free Radical that Vitamin C has no effect on.

The capability to eliminating oxygenation fat is much higher than that of Vitamin E

2.Toxicological experiment

Though serious of test on small mice, Tianxian Liquid has passed strict experiment on acute toxicity test, marrow cells micro test, germ cell aberration test and Ames test, also passed safety test for medicine toxicity.

3.Immunity function test

Though serious of test on small mice, to test:

1)Tianxian Liquid can enhance the protective ability for white blood cell

2)Enhance Lymph transformation in spleen greatly

3)Enhance hemolysis mechanism of blood serum and ability of anti-host of parasite, which can be understood as obviously improving immunity characteristics.

4.Restrain function for tumour

It can be demonstrated via small mice experiment on caruncle and liver cancer that the restrain function is not in the shade of chemical medicine 5-Fu;

And the more dosage used, the better effect of restrain can be obtained.

In addition, though comparative test with glossy ganoderma and green algae, Tianxian Liquid has obviously better effect than the comparative group.

Four experiment tests mentioned above can prove that Tianxian Liquid has already passed general scientific test.

Contact Information

Japan Branch of International Cancer Rehabilitation Association

Wang Zhenguo Office, Japan

102-0084 東京都千代田區二番町1 千代田

TEL: 03-5210 2246

FAX: 03 5210 4999

Monday -Friday

10:00 AM ---6:00 PM

Homepage Address: http://www.tensen.com

METAL出版

METAL Publishing

Home Page Mail- Address

E-mail : all@metamor.co.jp

Cured your diseases whatever situation has happened.

PART 2

One hundred cancer survivors' heart-warming and amazing stories

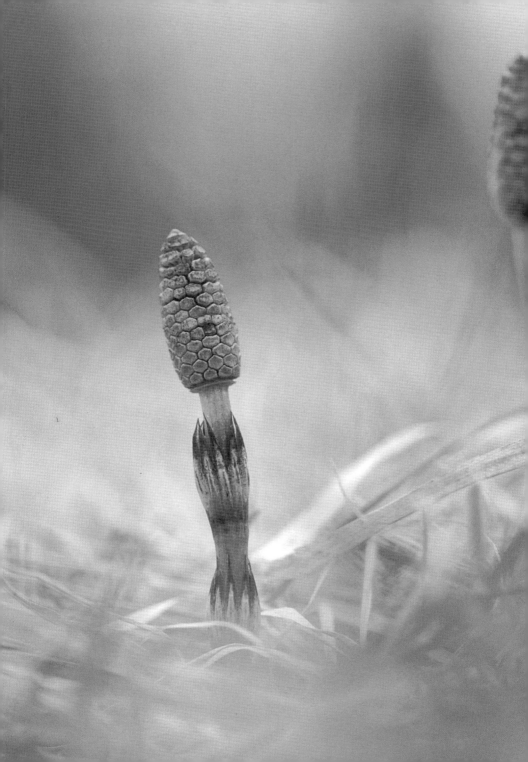

Experiences of defeating uterus cancer and breast cancer successfully

Defeat the monster of cancer twice

Edith Shih   San Francesco U.S.A. housewife 49

Do not "why I suffer from cancer ?"

Eight years ago my family immigrated to U.S.A. and were generally adapted to life there. My mother-in-law died of cancer, so I took care of the food and kept a balance of activities. In my regular and normal life, in October, 1997, I found that my physiological cycle was in disorder and felt lasting tiredness. After the examination at gynaecology department, I was diagnosed as suffering from "uterus cancer"

"Why did cancer catch me ?"

It was like a bolt from blue to know the result of the examination. When I was told to have only 5 years' survival, I made up my mind to try various kinds of treatment. From doctors' cold and mechanic tone, I felt that I was no longer a normal person but "a cancer patient". I felt deeply that "the so-called cancer patients are the target mechanically treated in the medical system".

I did not totally accept what doctors said. I made up my mind to have a thorough understanding of my disease before deciding on treatment, since it was I who would undergo the forthcoming treatment and defeat the disease. Tears could not solve the problem. After I calmed down, I began to collect information.

I decided on the ring-like taper-shaped operation on cervix of uterus. Since the cancer was detected at the early stage, it is not necessary to cut the whole uterus. Uterus is the most important organs of women, so I thought the uterus should be kept in any way. However, the doctor insisted on cutting away the whole uterus and ovary "to prevent the transfer". After listening to the doctor's suggestion, I became more firm that since I had only 5 years' survival, I should keep my uterus. From then on, my fighting against cancer began!

However, shortly afterwards, a serious event happened. The part which was going to be operated on bled terribly suddenly and could not be stopped. I drove to hospital at once. When I retrospect that event now, it seems as if God were blessing me, because all the traffic lights turned green on my way to the hospital. Normally it takes 25 minutes to the hospital, but on that day it took only 15 minutes in the rush hour.

The doctor at the hospital was surprised, " the degree of bleeding needs to call an ambulance!". I saw the seat in the car was covered with blood. Immediately I received an operation to treat the hurt. If I had arrived 5 minutes late, I would have died. Although I felt myself very lucky, the feeling of uneasiness was hanging over me. After the event, I began to take Tian Xian liquid in the middle of January, 1998.

One month later, in the middle of February, I returned to my hometown Taipei to spend the Spring Festival. The doctors there said that "it is not necessary to cut away the whole uterus and ovary", but to receive follow-up examination and various kinds of treatment. After returning to U.S.A., the doctor in charge and consultative doctor said that "operation is not necessary" too. I felt relieved eventually. There were many chances that I expressed my opinions through media and seminar to share my experiences with cancer patients.

Negligence led to another attack of cancer

However, after a period of time, cancer attacked me unexpectedly. In June, I felt myself fully recovered, so I had a trip to Southeast Asia with my family members. Maybe it was because I had eaten a lot of seafood like shrimps and crabs and hot food that had a bad effect on cancer during the trip that I suddenly suffered from the pain in joints of my feet and felt tired when we left for Japan in August. After returning to U.S.A., things did not improve. At an examination in November, the doctor found that there was a hard lump in my right breast. I remembered that 3 years, I found a hard lump in my breast, which disappeared after I took traditional Chinese medicine. I thought it was the same problem this time. But to be more cautious, I decided to have further check. Out of my expectation, the doctor's diagnosis is "breast cancer"! I regretted not taking Tian Xian liquid regularly and taking care in eating since I had thought that health had been restored. However, the series of attacks taught me a lesson in fighting against cancer!

Subsequently, the doctor put forward two suggestions: cutting away part of the breast (including lymph-vessels) and undergoing radiation treatment or cutting the whole breast. A doctor of traditional Chinese medicine said that cutting the whole breast would cause great damage to the Jingluo and therefore have influence on the whole body and suggested cutting part of the

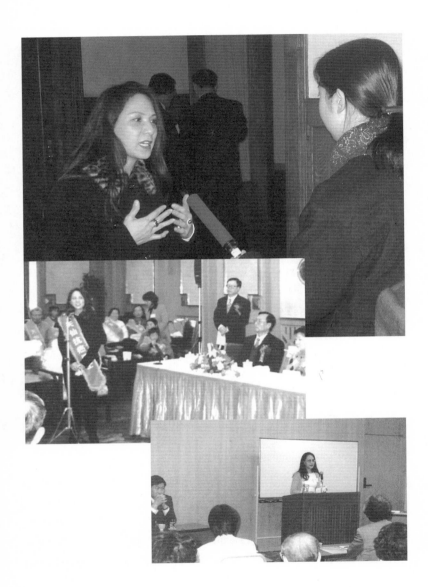

breast. After having an idea of the situation like last time, I chose to have part of the breast cut. I went to hospital in April, 1999 and received the operation to have part of the right breast cut away, a tumor of 2.5 cm taken out and lymph nodes under the right armpit cleared. Although I began to drink Tian Xian liquid immediately after the operation, I was unable to fall asleep because of tiredness after I went home. I felt that the vital energy of my body stagnant. So I applied Tian Xian plaster and slept till next morning.

One month later I began to receive radiation treatment. During this period, I felt increasing weak because of the side effects. To prevent transfer, I had my shoulder to abdomen irradiated by radioactive rays. I felt pain about my liver then lungs! Since my air tube was originally very weak, I became breathless and coughed terribly. Eventually, I even felt pain in kidney.

Grasp the critical moment and never give up easily

Looking back on the process of treatment, I had received radiation treatment 33 times all together. Suffering from the tremendous pain of treatment, I decided to use Tian Xian pills and Tian Xian plaster and went to nearby clinics of traditional Chinese medicine to receive massotheraphy on Jingluo. I felt that the side-effects were lessening, and my appetite was recovered and life began to be full of vitality. " I should be strong for family members and for myself!" Inspired by the strong will power, I completed the treatment successfully and returned to normal life.

First of all, we should be cautious in choosing the kinds of treatment, especially those that will not do harm to the whole body. We should try to regard operation as part of the treatment and combine other treatments to reduce the harm done to the body. Once the reproductive organ is cut away, hormone will be in imbalance. As a result, besides living the remaining life with hormone, other parts of the body such as bladder, large intestine, ureter will have problems one by one. That's why I insisted on keeping the uterus and ovary, since I knew that many women couldn't have their body restored to normal and even lose confidence after losing their reproductive organ.

Therefore, I appeal to avoid the treatment that will lead to the heavy burden of the body so as to reduce the damage to the minimum. Second, remember that re-attack or transfer is most likely to occur when the immunity is at the lowest level. As to me, cancer attacked me again because of tiredness and disorder of life during the trip. So it is very important to maintain a

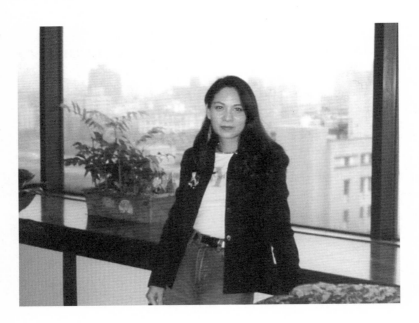

normal and regular life.

Third, pay attention to diet. Avoid certain food. Do not eat what should not be eaten. Control the amount of meat and fat. It is best to eat five cereals, beans, vegetable and keep a balanced diet.

Fourth, adjust emotions. After I knew that I suffered from cancer, I looked upon it as a chance to introspect life.

Since I am trying to do everything best, I always feel under pressure. But when the disease catches you, it is not what a perfectionist is able to control. So introspect your personality and let you have a thorough change.

No one can be perfect. But after making efforts, I find that I have become much more agreeable and gentle than before.

The last and the most important is to defeat cancer together with the love and support of family members. I remember that on the second day before the second operation, I came back from the hospital to find my husband weeping alone in darkness. I asked him, "what's the matter with you?" " Mother died of cancer. She was old. Although I felt sad, I still had to face life. But you are young. How could I live on without you⋯.", "I love you and I can't live without you. You can't be defeated anyway. You should live on for me⋯" Shedding tears, he uttered his sadness. My husband traveled in other places for his work and couldn't take care of me all the time. His tears strengthened my confidence of "regaining health for my husband and my children".

Now I am very healthy and live a happy life. Retrospecting that period, I can't help sighing with emotions, but I also obtained the most precious experiences in this way. No matter what diagnosis is, even if doctors can't help, you should never feel in despair. Never give up and hope will come. I fight with everyone with the determination of "never giving up"!

Cherish gratitude in heart

Miss Shimada Tokyo unemployed 44

Familial cancer

I was found to suffer from uterus cancer after I once fainted because of anaemia and sent to hospital for an examination. That was May, 1995. The doctor said that the cancer was "at the third stage" and was progressive, and suggested an operation immediately. But I refused. Both my parents died of cancer, especially my mother who used to be plump but was reduced to skeleton after the operation and passed away soon.

I think I inherited the cancer factor from my parents. Besides, my immunity was overloaded because of my eating habit, mental and physical pressure and environmental problem. Thus, cancer attacked me. Afterwards, I began to collect information and search for treatment suitable for me. I found it was necessary to adjust the steps of life besides changing eating habit.

I was managing a small company and very busy at that time. My sleeping and diet were not regular. Therefore, I decided to resign the job. As to diet, I preferred meat and ate chafing dish and Japanese beef dish in turn day by day. Now I think what triggered off cancer was eating a large amount of meat every day. Thus, now I eat brown rice, vegetable (root and leaf) and seaweed as the main food.

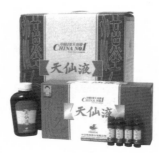

Improve my physique to take in the medicine fully

The most important thing is to improve immunity. Besides, Tian Xian liquid, Tian Xian pills and Tian Xian plaster, I have tried all that help improve immunity like acupuncture and moxibustion, finger-press, Korean herbs and natural health tea from Brazil.

However, even I took Tian Xian liquid and to take as much as nutrition as possible, but the digestive system did not work well, not only unable to take in nutrition but even unable to excrete harmful substances. In order to enhance the function of the digestive system, I began to try a plum essence (梅精) diet. On the other hand, for nutrition to be sent to every part of the body, I began to put my feet in hot water for some time to enhance the circulation of blood.

With such effort, the physical and mental status did not give cancer cells the chance to spread and the effects of medicine appeared. I had been diagnosed as suffering from cancer of IIIb stage, but when I was reexamined the next year, the cancer cells seemed to be disappearing, although I was not recovered thoroughly. It was because I began to know how to keep myself in a happy mood after I was found to suffer from cancer. The reason why I could fight against cancer is that I always keep myself happy and cherish gratitude to all people and things. I once travelled abroad and even forgot that I suffered from "an incurable disease".

The irregular life and pressure caused the increase of dangerous factors during the 10 years and therefore triggered off cancer. So I should fight 10 more years to eliminate cancer thoroughly. To achieve this goal, I should be confident and maintain the present state of life. I am sure we can prevent transfer and another attack of cancer only if we change living habit, maintain the environment favorable for treatment so as not to let the cancer cells spread.

137

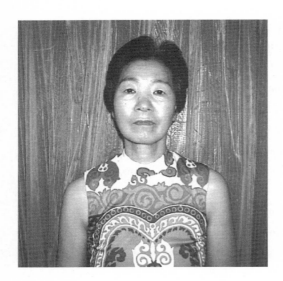

Value the remaining life more

Lady Nakagawa Osaka housewife 62

Diagnosed as cystitis by mistake

At first, I felt uncomfortable suddenly. That was July, 1998. I felt piercing pain around my hips. So I went to hospital and was diagnosed as "cystitis".

After several months' treatment in hospital, the pain was not reduced but enhanced. Finally I abdomen began to swell and it was difficult to walk.

After ECHO examination, the doctor was convinced that I had serious ascites. Thus, I was rushed to a big hospital equipped with modern facilities. Out of my expectation, the diagnosis was ovary cancer, and I could live for only 6 months. Since the tumor had increased to 12 cm, the operation was impossible and I had to rely on chemical treatment.

At that time, my daughter found a book entitled "Fighting against Cancer". She believed the experience described in the book and bought Tian Xian liquid for me immediately. I began to take 8 small bottles of the liquid (80cc) every day and continued for several months. It was so unbelievable that when I went to hospital for another examination, the tumor was reduced to half the size. The doctor opened his eyes wide, " perhaps the operation can be performed." Several months later, the doctor performed the operation as planned before.

I had my ovary, uterus and caecum cut away, for cancer was suspected to have transferred to these parts. Later the doctor announced that my tumor disappeared completely. I remember that I was able to go to the toilet by myself the second day after the examination. Even the nurses were surprised. I was also surprised at my quick recovery. I believe all this is attributed to Tian Xian liquid.

I was released from hospital shortly afterwards. Now I go 'to hospital to have an examination every Tuesday. Besides, in order to prevent another attack of cancer, I continue to take Tian Xian liquid. I am 62 years old now and I will value the remaining life more.

Pursue the beautiful life when suffering from a disease beyond cure

Miss Sato   Miyazaki county   housewife 36

Lucky to escape from death

Two years ago I was diagnosed as suffering from cancerous pleurisy transferred from ovary cancer. The treatment plan was to undergo an operation to have the ovary cancer cut away after the physical status was bettered. Before the operation, I should receive chemical treatment.

However, all the anti-cancer drugs were had no effect. At that time, my physical status was bad and I had almost no appetite. The X-rays found something in two sides of the chest and tumor and something in the right ovary. The doctor said that the situation was very serious. When the disease continued to aggravate, a friend told me that someone recovered from ovary cancer of the second stage by taking traditional Chinese medicine, which was exactly Tian Xian liquid. Thus I bought Tian Xian liquid immediately and began to drink it.

After taking Tian Xian liquid for half a year, I resumed my appetite and my physical status improved. I was quite different from my former self and could even be released from hospital. The tumor in ovary did not change much, but the something in my chest reduced and that in my abdomen disappeared completely.

I continue to take Tian Xian liquid after returning home from hospital. Although I haven't recovered from cancer, I am still in the pursuit of the beautiful life with cancer existing in my body. I'd like to thank Tian Xian liquid for helping me enjoy life again.

A beam of light in darkness

Lau Siu Ying Hong Kong housewife 65

Cancer attacked me again together with transfer; I was thrown in great despair

I was first found to suffer from uterus cancer in 1996. Part of the uterus and ovary were cut away for my old age to prevent transfer.

After the operation, I received radiation treatment to prevent transfer. In the spring of 1997, cancer cells were found in the remaining part of the uterus and even transferred to chest and brain! After I was examined and treated painfully in hospital for some time, doctors were still unable to control the attack of cancer. The inability of the doctors threw me in despair. They said nothing but anti-cancer drugs and radiation treatment might be of some help to me. But I'd rather suffer the pain than receive meaningless treatment.

When I was in despair, Doctor Wang Zhengguo whom my elder brother knew raised the suggestion of "taking Tian Xian liquid continuously for half a year" and others after having an idea of my condition. I was excited at the suggestion. Shortly after taking the medicine under his instructions, I felt my appetite and physical status improved. Six months after taking Tian Xian liquid, no one could discern that I suffer from cancer. Even doctors were surprised at my quick recovery.

Afterwards, I went to hospital once a month for regular examination. The diagnosis is that the transferred tumor has almost disappeared and the tumor in the uterus has disappeared subsequently.

Living is the best proof

Liang Bai Cuizhu Taiwan Taipei housewife 62

I took Tian Xian liquid alone and cancer cells disappeared

At first, my weight dropped from 50km to 45 km out of no reason. My daughter was worried for me and accompanied me to Tai Da Hospital for examination. Out of my expectation, the doctor told me that I suffer from uterus cancer of the third stage.

I was in hospital for half a year to receive chemical treatment. During that period of time, my daughter heard that her friend's husband suffered from stomach cancer and could live only half a year, but he recovered for taking Tian Xian liquid. So she suggested me taking Tian Xian liquid too. After I was released from hospital, I began to take Tian Xian liquid.

At the beginning, I drank 4 bottles of the liquid per day and continued for 8 days, then 3 bottles per day and continued one year and two months. Recently, after the examination, the doctor was surprised to find that cancer cells disappeared completely in my body.

I did not tell him about Tian Xian liquid for doctors in Taiwan believe that Chinese ways of treatment do not work at all. I did not want to hurt his self-esteem. But it is the fact that I do defeat cancer. So I suggest other patients taking Tian Xian liquid.

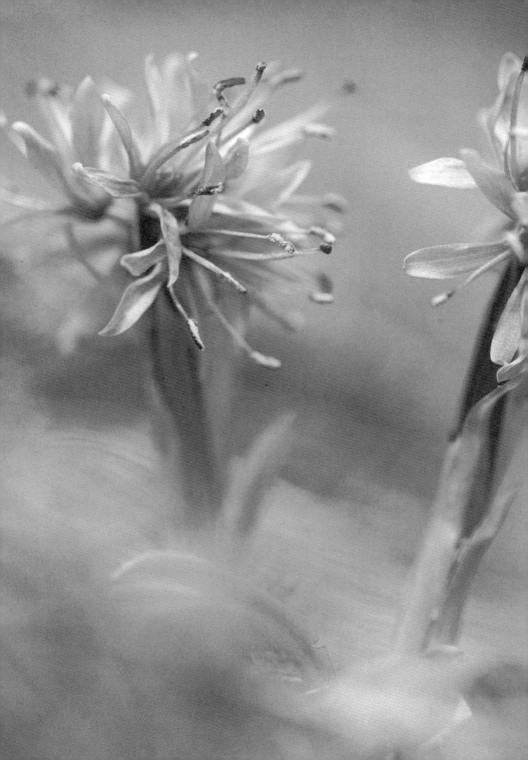

Experiences of defeating breast cancer successfully

Gain the courage in the embrace of nature

Lady Okada Gifu County housewife 69

Cancer attacked again out of negligence

My family manages a hot spring hotel that has been passed on for several generations. My youngest son and his wife are in charge of the hotel. As we prepared to enjoy the leisure life after retiring, my husband underwent an operation for stomach disease in November, 1986. Since then, together with other diseases, my husband has had to seek medical help every day for 13 years.

My husband began to take Tian Xian liquid from 1990. At that time, I was suffering from breast cancer and had my left breast cut away. So my husband suggested me taking Tian Xian liquid together to prevent another attack. For these years, I have not caught serious diseases and there has no sign of another attack. But I have not taken Tian Xian liquid seriously.

In the regular examination in May, 1999, the doctor found cancer cells in my right breast and decided on and operation. Thanks to the early detection, the disease had not developed out of control. Then I began to take Tian Xian liquid seriously. Later, I was sent to hospital for the great side-effects of anti-cancer drugs. When I was in hospital, I insisted on taking Tian Xian liquid behind the doctor's back. After one year, I resumed my strength. But I do not help in the hotel now but concentrate all my attention on floriculture besides housework.

Several days ago, I took part in the local gathering. When people saw me in high spirit, they said, " you do not look like a cancer patient at all." It is so marvelous for one who had cancer in the two breasts successively.

We live in Ao Fei Chan, where there is the most beautiful nature. The mountains are covered with green in summer and with white snow in winter. Appreciating the changing seasons, my heart is in the state of peace and tranquility. In such beautiful environment, I was filled with the courage to fight against cancer.

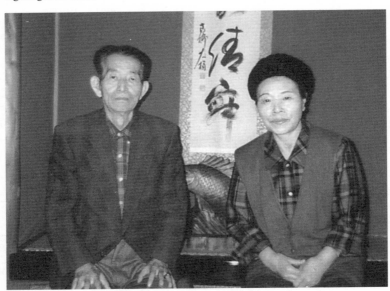

Regain vitality and hope

Lady Nakada   Osaka   housewife   59

Cruel tortures came one after another

Four years ago, mother suffered from breast cancer. At that time, the tumor was 5 cm in size and had transferred to the lymph gland. She was injected with anti-cancer drugs immediately after the operation. About one year later, the tumor in another breast was reduced and it was time to cut away part of the breast and receive radiation treatment. However, the torture inflicted on mother did not stop. Two years later, cancer cells were found in the lymph glands under the throat. The doctor told us that mother could live for only one or two years.

At that time, elder brother saw some information on Tian Xian liquid on internet. Frankly speaking, after reading the detailed account, we did not have much trust in it, because we had tried numerous anti-cancer secret prescriptions, but all of them were of no effect. So had thought that Tian Xian liquid was only one of them.

However, what was the most serious was that the treatment in hospital achieved no effect at all. Mother grew very weak as a result of the serious side-effects and said in disappointment, "it is meaningless to continue the treatment." I felt deeply grieved. Then I thought of Tian Xian liquid and placed an order immediately. I let mother drink it 20 days before the sixth injection of anti-cancer drug. The effect was obvious. The tumor near the lymph gland was reduced in size! Then I decided to stop the treatment of anti-cancer drugs and keep a close eye on the subsequent development.

Four months later, the tumor has not increased nor reduced in size. But mother is very vigorous. Although she has not fully recovered, I am convinced that Tian Xian liquid is the only one that can fight against cancer. I hope that all the other patients suffering from cancer like mother can have an understanding of Tian Xian liquid and take it as soon as possible.

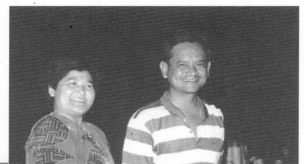

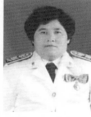

Enjoy the happiness of life again

Lady Saho Thailand teacher 45

Bedridden because of side-effects

In the physical examination 7 years ago, cancer cells were found in the right breast. Operation followed then. Two years later, the cancer cells were transferred to the left breast and I underwent another operation. To prevent another attack I received anti-drug treatment twice and radiation treatment 50 times.

Although both radiation and anti-cancer drug could control cancer cells, the side-effects were inevitable. I felt great pain in my whole body, dazed, and even had difficulty in walking. I had to be bedridden, taken care of by others, let alone work.

In December 1999, I saw the introduction of Tian Xian liquid on TV. I immediately place an order by phone before the TV show ended. After taking the liquid for a month, I felt my strength was enhanced, the unbearable side-effects were reduced and my appetite returned to normal.

Several months later, examination showed that my body was recovered and I could walk around by myself. Recently besides teaching, I began to take MBA courses in holiday. At present, my strength, health and complexion are no different from that of normal people. I think I can recover better!

Now every time I hear that someone suffers from cancer, I will immediately introduce Tian Xian liquid to them. Readers , do not misunderstand me as promoting the sale. I only hope that other cancer patients who suffer the tremendous pain from anti-cancer drugs and radiation treatment can recover health with the help of Tian Xian liquid.

Regain life with the blessing of God

Lady Alina Philippines Manila housewife 53

Insist on refusing operation

In June, 1997, I went to complex hospital in Manila to have an examination on chest. Out of my expectation, the doctor told me that I suffered from breast cancer and said in a sincere tone, "there is still the possibility of treatment and the radiation treatment will begin on Monday." Before I went home, I prayed in the small church in the hospital, very worried. After I returned home, I couldn't help weeping and my family members tried hard to suppress their sorrow and prayed with me.

Although treatment followed immediately, I still expected that I did not suffer from breast cancer. So I went to other hospitals to undergo examination. Unfortunately, all hospitals expressed unanimously, "we are sure that you have breast cancer. It is in the preliminary stage, you'd better have chemical treatment." No matter how firmly I refused to undergo an operation, the doctor still insisted on the necessity of an operation and the sooner, the better.

When I was in such a dilemma, my husband went back with Tian Xian liquid.

It was in October. After taking Tian Xian liquid for a week, I obviously felt the hard lump in the breast softening gradually. Several days later, some pus-like substance broke from under the skin, then blood flowed out. Up till December, the 1.25-inch hard lump disappeared but bleeding did not stop. So I continued to take Tian Xian liquid.

In January, 1998, I was sent to hospital for losing consciousness. I underwent a medical examination after blood transfusion. It was found that cancer cells had disappeared! All this is so unbelievable!

More energetic than before

Wang Meiyun Malaysia housewife 41

A hard lump developed into breast cancer

At the end of 1999, I felt pain in the breast and went to hospital to undergo X-ray examination. The doctor's diagnosis was "there is a hard lump in the breast that deserves attention". As days went by, the pain was becoming more and more acute and the hard lump in the upper part on the left was increasing in size quickly. When I went to hospital for examination, the hard lump developed into breast cancer. Afterwards, under the doctor's instructions, I underwent an operation to have the breast cut away, the tumor taken out, received chemical and radiation treatment.

During this period, I suffered a lot from diarrhea, vomit, loss of appetite, reduction in weight, and dropping of hair, which were the side-effects of treatment. In March, 1997, a friend of my husband's, who was a doctor, got some information about Tian Xian liquid on internet and urged me to take it immediately. Three months later, I went to hospital for regular examination and the doctor said that the part that had been operated on was in normal condition and the lymph lump under the armpit disappeared. Drinking Tian Xian liquid mitigated the side-effects of chemical and radiation treatment. My appetite and strength recovered subsequently. I even found myself more energetic than what I was before catching the disease! What was the most exciting was that the hair had grown out.

To prevent another attack of cancer, I reduce the amount of Tian Xian liquid I take to 200 cc (2 bottles) every day. Now, regular examination every 3 months shows that "everything is normal". I finally understand what real health is. I will cherish my gratitude to Tian Xian liquid for ever.

The hint of death encourages fighting

Lady Ohara   Totori   County   housewife   43

Side-effects were mitigated immediately

It was in May that the examination showed a 5 cm large tumor in my left breast. After receiving chemical treatment for some time, I underwent an operation. Afterwards, I received chemical treatment again for 3 stages.

It is all due to reports about Tian Xian liquid my husband saw when I was in hospital that I am able to live on healthy. That was in the middle of June.

After taking Tian Xian liquid, I immediately felt that the side-effects of chemical treatment were mitigated. Vomiting and hair-dropping stopped. Besides, appetite recovered and the number of white blood cells did not reduce.

Doctors and nurses who did not know that I was taking Tian Xian liquid were surprised to say, " Mrs. Ohara is very special". At such effects, I decided to continue drink Tian Xian liquid. I will never forget that the doctor said, " another breast cancer patient of your age and in the same condition died about 2 months after leaving hospital. Maybe you have only two months to live. So ···" The doctor's vague hint " can you accept death?" did not depress me but encouraged me to fight instead. So I think I should thank him.

In fact, the role Tian Xian liquid plays is dramatic. I have drunk it for 2 years and the cancer does not transfer, nor deteriorates. Although it is still necessary to take Tian Xian liquid continulusly, I am able to do some housework, have a walk with family members outside and enjoy buying.

Live peacefully with cancer

Mr Gotou Tokushima County 49

Chinese friends brought my saviour

I was found to suffer from breast cancer in a medical examination 3 years ago. I underwent an operation immediately. The tumor was 1.5cm , but the doctor asked me not to worry because it was in the preliminary stage. In another examination shortly afterwards, the cancer was transferred to several parts in the bone. The diagnosis was that the cancer had developed into the fourth state and I could only live for one or two years.

After I was released from hospital, I did not want to be defeated by cancer and continued to work. At the same time, my husband and I were searching for medicine and treatment effective against cancer and received treatment in hospital.

One day, a Chinese friend brought Tian Xian liquid which he said was very effective against cancer. I drank it immediately. Out of my expectation, two and three days later, my strength improved and gradually recovered. From then on, I took Tian Xian liquid every day. It has been 3 years since the operation. Although cancer cells exist in several parts of my body, they do not grow, nor transfer.

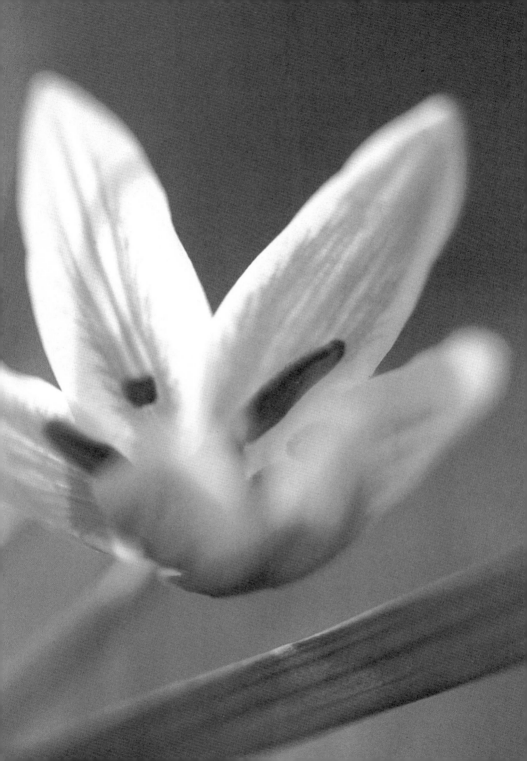

Experiences of defeating lung cancer successfully

A warrior who has fought against cancer for 10 years

Mr Fukuda Yamakuchi County jobless 68

Death approached once

My husband has fought against cancer for 10 years.

In 1990, he had his rectum and left kidney cut away. Afterwards, he was sent to hospital for cancer attacked pelvis near rectum. After repeated treatment of radiation, heat and anti-cancer drugs, the disease was under control. He received regular examination and took anti-cancer drugs.

At that time, we got to know Tian Xian liquid from reports. He tried drinking it from January, 1996 but did not take it seriously. In September, tumors of 5 to 10 cm were found in his two lungs and operation was impossible. In such worry, he bought and ate all that were said to be effective against cancer such as . One year later, in April, 1998, the tumors were found to have grown 2 to 5 cm larger. The doctor said that the patient should be immediately sent to hospital to receive the treatment of anti-cancer drugs, otherwise, he was dying soon. Thus, he was in hospital again.

My husband drank Tian Xian liquid and at the same time took anti-cancer drugs. I do not know if it was due to the combined the effect of the two that the side-effect my husband suffered seemed less than that of other patients. Stomatitis and diarrhea were not serious. And when he was released from hospital, the tumor even reduced to half the size. With the physical status improving, my husband who is always credulous heard that water soluble glucose was particularly effective against lung cancer. So he bought it and took it without second thought and stopped drinking Tian Xian liquid. However, at the end of 1998, he could not take in food, let alone taste it.

Anti-cancer traditional Chinese medicine took effect

In April, 1999, the cancer in pelvis attacked again. My husband grew increasingly weaker and was sent to hospital. The condition was very terrible at that time. the tumor pierced through his small intestine and excrement was released with urine and even with blood. He could not take in food for a month and a half and lived on drip feeding. In order to take in food, the doctor performed an operation on him to connect large intestine with small intestine. After he was released from hospital in June, 1999, he began to take Tian Xian liquid seriously, drinking 6 bottles per day plus Tian Xian pills.

In December, 1999, X-rays, blood test, ECHO examination showed that he was in good physical state except pneumonedema in the chest and signs of cancer. Another examination in January, 2000 showed that although the tumor in the lung did not change, pneumonedema in the chest was reduced in amount and the sign of tumor showed the tendency of being lowered. The doctor in charge was satisfied and asked, " have you taken some other medicine?" "yes, a traditional Chinese medicine." The doctor felt it unbelievable and was even

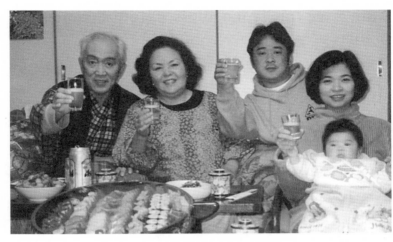

dumbfounded in amazement when he heard my husband say that he did not feel pain in the chest , no cough or phlegm.

Now, despite the lowering of tumor sign since the beginning of the year, cancer is found to have been transferred to the brain. My husband is in hospital for treatment now. Although he has not won the battle against cancer, he has escaped from death several times and keeps high spirit for fighting. We are convinced that he will recover. In good weather, I drive him to the suburb for a walk and even clime to the peak of the mountain and vow to fight against cancer together, "cancer, keep as far away as possible!". Anyway, we are fighting together. We have a plan that after he is released from hospital peacefully, we will have a trip to Shan Yang, enjoying the beautiful scenery and the brilliant life as usual.

Care from family members defeat the monster of cancer

Mr Kisohara Mie County company employee 69

The physical body of my son is in Tokyo but his heart is with me.

At first, the doctor announced that I could live only half a year. The tumor was at the bottom of the right lung near artery, with a size of 7cm x 6cm in the third stage. In the operation performeded in March, 1999, the tumor could not be cut away completely. So I had to undergo chemical and radiation treatment. It was in May when I was in hospital that I began to drink Tian Xian liquid. My youngest son who lives in Tokyo collected information on internet and believed Tian Xian liquid to be the most effective after his analysis.

After I took Tian Xian liquid, the side-effects were mitigated, I could taste the delicious food and my strength resumed. When I was released from hospital in June, the tumor was reduced to half the size. I continued to take Tian Xian liquid afterwards and the CT examinations in December last year and March this year did not find the trace of cancer cells. Now I am very energetic. I am active in gatherings and trips for the old and even participated in the regular meeting of directors last year. Many directors said that I looked refreshed.

Of course I should thank Tian Xian liquid for my recovery. But the people I owe the most gratitude to are my son and my wife, especially my son who lives in Tokyo but is much concerned about me and reminds me to take Tian Xian liquid constantly.

To cure my disease my son's is filled with books about cancer. Besides Tian Xian liquid, he also told me various other treatments. I am proud of my son who is so much concerned about me besides his busy work. I will fight against cancer courageously to live up to my wife and son's care and great efforts.

"Confidence" is the only road to cure

Mr Eta   Yamaguchi County jobless 72

I was negligent out of over-confidence

Anyone can catch cancer but we don't know why? In the spring of 1998, I went to hospital to have regular X-ray examination on chest for high blood pressure. A shadow was found on my left lung. But I did not feel anything abnormal about myself so I just ignored it. In November, 1998, the doctor suggested me having a medical examination in hospital. Out of my expectation, the result showed that it was lung cancer. The doctor suggested operation and chemical treatment. But the operation was difficult because my respiratory function was weak and the cancer was near the artery. Finally I decided to undergo chemical treatment. The doctor told me that chemical treatment would result in side-effects like loss of appetite, vomiting, diarrhea, hair-dropping. Therefore, I must store as much strength as possible to cope with chemical treatment.

I bought two kinds of heal food and hid it from the doctor. During this period, my wife tried her best to collect various sorts of information about health food and traditional Chinese medicine.

In the process of chemical treatment, no other side-effects appeared except hair-dropping. When I was released from hospital in March, 1999, the tumor was reduced in size but still existed. I made up my mind to wipe it out thoroughly. So I tried to search for other good medicines.

I firmly believed the anti-cancer effects of traditional Chinese medicine.

According to past experiences, I believed that traditional Chinese medicine was only cure for cancer, because it works in a milder way than western medicine and can help improve immunity. At that time, I found the book entitled "Fighting against Cancer". After reading it carefully, I was convinced that this was the traditional Chinese medicine I need. Thus, I drank 4 bottles of the liquid every day.

Now, I not only have a good appetite, but also put on weight. At my improvement, relatives and friends said, "the diagnosis of cancer may be a mistake!" The postman who delivers Tian Xian liquid regularly per month asked me curiously who was the patient for he knew that the medicine is for cancer. When I told him it was me, he could not cover his astonishment.

Although the cancer has not disappeared completely, it shows no sign of transfer. The doctor says that it is not necessary to continue the treatment. I do not seem to have disease although there is the focus in my body. So I believe even the focus will disappear one day. I began to collect information about the treatment and medicine for cancer after I was told to suffer from cancer. The deeper understanding I have of cancer, the more hope I get. Thus , I think that believing "I will recover soon" and the effect of medicine will bring life to me. This is the most important link of curing cancer.

I believe this is what I need most.

Snatch the last straw

Mr Kitahara Osaka responsible personnel of a company 45

The shadow after 7 years

In the cold early spring of February, 1999, my elder brother had a fall when he was checking the construction on site and had his rib broken. Although he recovered, but serious fact followed. Seven years, he underwent an operation to have 4/5 of his stomach cut away. He was worried about the transfer but did not mention it to relatives and friends. However, a shadow was found in the X-ray examination on chest.

Since he did not feel anything abnormal about himself, doctors decided keep an eye on it at first. Days passed. At the end of the season, when shoots appeared on twigs, brother suddenly felt piercing pain in the back.

At first he thought the pain was in the muscle. But it grew to be acute. Finally an ambulance was called to send him to hospital. Since the cause of the unbearable pain is unknown, another examination on chest was carried out. The pain might be the initial abnormality or felt symptom. The diagnosis was like a bolt from the blue. It was "lung cancer" and had been transferred to bone! The operation was so difficult and was given up.

Never to be defeated by cancer

"Why is there no symptom when the disease has developed to such a serious degree?" "Why is operation difficult?" What was more unacceptable was that "he could only live for 2 years"! I still clearly remember the sorrow, despair, panic of all people at that time and dare not look back. We decided not to let brother know his disease.

After the examination, treatment began, including radiation treatment for 30 times, anti-cancer drug treatment for 3 times (3 stages). Since he was sent to hospital, I called him every day. "I may have caught cancer." From the other end of the line came brother's calm voice. I tried my best to speak in a calm tone, "don't worry, brother. You are sure to recover." Such words seem to give me more courage. My elder sister who tried her best to suppress the sorrow encouraged him, "never to be defeated by cancer. You must have the confidence in recovery and not disappoint us."

I believed there must be good cure and vowed to find it. Thus, I searched medical academies or cancer hospitals for information. The more I knew, the more helpful for the treatment. Finally, I found Tian Xian liquid which had actual effects on cancer. I called the Japanese branch of International Cancer Recovery Association in excitement. Getting the document, I told brother immediately, "I have found the medicine that is sure to cure cancer".

I took Tian Xian liquid and Tian Xian pills that I bought to hospital. As brother was to drink it, the doctor in charge said that it was not allowed to take other anti-cancer medicine except those provided by the hospital. So we had to give it up temporarily in hospital. However, brother suffered a great deal from the side-effects (reduction in the number of white blood cells, fever, loss of appetite, physical weakness) of chemical and radiation treatment. He said, "I'd rather die than bear such sufferings!" I only hoped that brother could leave hospital and take Tian Xian liquid. Eventually, the treatment in hospital finished and brother could leave hospital after several examinations were done.

However, the result of the examinations threw everyone into despair. "No improvement. Cancer cells have not disappeared," said the doctor.

Then, what was the use of the treatment that caused so great and painful side-effects? Traditional Chinese medicine was not allowed and the doctor's instructions should be followed. But what about the result? No one present could say something for extreme sorrow. But I didn't believe the result of the examination and I vowed to myself, "we can't trust doctors any more. Brother will lose his life if we do not take other measures. I should try my best to save my brother's life." As soon as brother left hospital, I let him drink Tian Xian liquid. Afterwards, he drank Tian Xian liquid 6 times and took Tian Xian pills 3 times a day (9 pills at first). On the second day after brother came back, he began to have a walk around. At first, he was out of breath and unstable in walking. However, 4 days after he took Tian Xian products, everyone could see sign of his recovering. He was no longer breathless after walk, his appetite turned good, his weight increased and the complexion became ruddy. In order to confirm whether brother's recovery was due to the function of Tian Xian products, I went to consult the doctor if anti-cancer drugs still worked on patients like brother who stopped the treatment for some time. The answer was "impossible". after walking out of the hospital, I was to exclaim at the effects of Tian Xian liquid. In September, the first examination after brother left hospital realized our dream. The tumor was obviously reduced in size and it was only 1 month since brother began to take Tian Xian liquid! In another examination one month later, since it was necessary to take anti-cancer drugs, the doctor suggested my brother living in hospital for care.

Although we did not fully trust the treatment in hospital, we could not make the right judgement by ourselves but to accept the doctor's instructions. A few days after brother was in hospital, he again lost his appetite, unable to take in food, even the fruit to complement vitamins. He was weaker than before when he left hospital 3 weeks later. In October, he stopped taking anti-cancer drugs, but Tian Xian pills and Tian Xian liquid. But I still kept contact with hospitals and doctors I trust and told them that we could not accept the treatment that led to the loss of appetite.

Enjoy the happiness of life again

In November, I sought help from a professor from a hospital of a university. We showed him the medical record from the first hospital and the result of examination from another hospital. After his detailed explanation, we were surprised that the isotope examination did not show anything abnormal and the bone to which cancer transferred turned normal. X-ray and CT examination showed that cancer cells were going to be eliminated completely. At that time, brother had taken Tian Xian liquid for 3 months. In December when Christmas was approaching, the city was enveloped in an atmosphere of coming festival. Brother went to the hospital of the university for medical check once a month. Every time the professor looked at the CT picture, he could not help smiling and said, "very good. It's better to keep an eye on it to prevent another attack." My brother who could not suppress his happiness asked the professor, "can I drink wine?" He was overjoyed.

The examination in January and February, 2000 showed that even the sign of tumor turned normal, cancer cells disappeared completely and physical strength was resumed. My hardworking brother has returned to his post and looks energetic every day.

I'd like to express my sincerest gratitude to every member at the Japanese branch of International Cancer Recovery Association and Mr. Wang who have encouraged for the year and the God who is always blessing us! I also hope that all cancer patients take Tian Xian liquid as soon as possible, find reliable doctors and never give up!

Forget the disease and live a vigorous life

Mr. Yang Taiwan Taipei housewife 71

My mother-in-law is open to the outside world even when suffering from disease

My mother-in-law who used to work on site when she was young can't live without doing anything. She either weaves sweaters and others or rides her bicycle around. She didn't go to school because in childhood of poverty, so she attends evening class at present. Besides, she is a voluntary worker for her life. My mother-in-law is so energetic and healthy that she had almost never caught disease. However, in October 1998, she suddenly coughed out bloody phlegm. The medical examination showed that she suffered from lung cancer and it was at the final stage.

I have not told the fact to her.

After she underwent an operation and was released from hospital, my husband heard his friends talk about a good traditional Chinese medicine. Thus, she began to take Tian Xian liquid from December.

Tian Xian liquid took effect quickly and my mother-in-law has gradually recovered to the original "energetic mother". She once said, " the chance to contact the outside world can not be given up even if one has caught disease."

I did not what to do before, but now I encourage my mother-in-law to do whatever she wants to do. Although fate is beyond control, we must live a vigorous life to the end.

The fortunes and misfortunes of life are unpredictable

Lady Nakamura Tokyo housewife 62

The threat of transfer was hanging over me

I have always been confident of my health. But out of my expectation, in 1994, the doctor announced that I had breast cancer and cut away the whole of my right breast. Afterwards, I began to take hormone medicine and stopped two years later.

In April, 1999, two examinations per year showed that the cancer transferred to the lung. Tomography suggested that cancer cells were in the shape of spore and there were something in the chest. The doctor said that both the operation and radiation were impossible. In June, after the treatment of anti-cancer drugs for 3 times, almost all my hair had dropped. Although there was nothing wrong with my body, I was under extreme mental pressure. I was so worried at the doctors' perfunctory treatment of anti-cancer drugs and hormone to the "possible transfer". Restlessly, I had to rely on myself to seek relevant information for treatment.

Since I believed that "cancer research originated in China" and my husband's brother recommended the book "Fighting against Cancer", I immediately took Tian Xian liquid and Tian Xian pills. In September, X-ray check showed that the result was satisfactory and the tumor sign lowered to 45. Both the doctor and I were surprised at the fact. However, since I tried several other medicines and stopped Tian Xian liquid, consequently the tumor sign rose up to 49. To prevent the aggravation, I began to take Tian Xian liquid and Tian Xian pills from 24th, November.

In January this year, tumor sign dropped to 44 again. After tomography, the doctor was convinced that "there is no cancer cell". Shortly afterwards, the tumor sign returned normal.

Now, the dropped hair have grown on my head and physical and mental state returned normal. I always think " if there were no Tian Xian liquid" or " I had caught cancer 10 years ago", everything would be different.

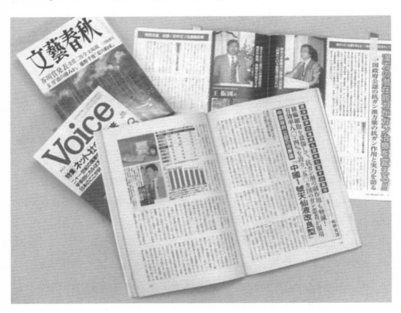

Smell the air of twenty first century with my wife

Lady Yamane Fukushima County housewife 55

Modern medicine could not help

In November, 1999, my wife went to hospital for examination because of the great pain in shoulder. The doctor announced that there was a tumor of 1.5 cm at the lower part of right lung. Since it was discovered early, there was not danger of death if the tumor was cut away. In December when my wife and I waited for the operation at home, the doctor in charge of the operation asked me to go to the hospital.

He explained to me that " although the primary cancer is small, but is malignant to a high degree and has been transferred to other parts." Finally he said, "there is at most one year to live." At this news, I felt dazed, almost dropping to the ground. After the operation, my wife received the treatment of anti-cancer drugs. But it had to be stopped because of the unbearable pain she suffered from. Besides, radiation treatment is only effective on certain features of the cancer. The doctor said in disappointment that even modern medicine could not help.

But I could not give up. I began to search for various kinds of prescriptions, collect health magazines and information from advertisements in newspapers. I let my wife try all medicines that are effective against cancer such as shark paste, AHCC. So since I got to know books about Tian Xian liquid, I bought it for my wife without hesitation.

From then on, my wife stays away from side-effects and is even able to have a trip.

In fact, I did not tell the real condition of the disease to my wife but only said that it was to prevent transfer and another attack. My wife also waited to see the effects of Tian Xian liquid and took it regularly. However, she caught a terrible cold in November last year, which led to water accumulation in the right lung, and was sent to hospital again. At the beginning of this year, she could not take in food nor sleep for the great pain in the part on which the operation was performed and in the back, and had to rely on morphine to stop the pain. The further examination showed that the cancer cells had transferred to ribs, which caused the pain. Seeing my wife inflicted by the pain, my spiritual sufferings were beyond description in human language.

Now, we can only expect the effects of Tian Xian liquid and hope that my wife can smell the air of twenty first century with my wife.

It is not a dream to restore life to normal

Mr Nakashima Tokyo jobless 74

A right decision

At first, CT examination on chest showed something abnormal. It was confirmed to be cancer after more precise check. Treatment followed immediately. That was in September, 1999. On the bus that took me to hospital, I saw the advertisement for the book "Fight against Cancer". After reading the book carefully, I decided to try Tian Xian liquid.

173

I contacted the Japanese branch of International Cancer Recovery Association and began to take Tian Xian liquid under their instructions. Two months later, I clearly felt that my strength was improving. The subsequent examination showed that the cancer did not grow. Besides, my appetite recovered and complexion turned ruddy. The doctor said that I could feel relieved.

The examination conducted at the beginning of the year showed that the tumor sign (CEA) was 39. I think I can resume my normal life. The effects of Tian Xian liquid will be more obvious some time later. I will make more efforts and at the same time hope that other patients can all accept Tian Xian.

Family members' support is the best cure

Zhu Cheng Taiwan Taipei jobless 66

The son gave up learning abroad for father

174

At first, my husband was always out of breath when he climbed the stairs. I had not suspected that it was the initial sign. In May, 1998, the doctor diagnosed that he suffered from "lung cancer" at the late stage.

Then my husband received the treatment of anti-cancer drug, but the side-effects like vomiting were very serious and he became weak. After he received treatment of traditional Chinese medicine in Shanghai last September, the condition improved temporarily but deteriorated immediately. When we were at a loss what to do, we were lucky enough to know of Tian Xian liquid. Convinced that it can really improve immunity, I decided to put my husband's life into the hands of Tian Xian liquid.

He began to take 6 bottles of Tian Xian liquid, 3 bottles of natural nutritious liquid which belong to Tian Xian series and Tian Xian paste. Three months later, the medicine took obvious effect. Althoug he was still breathless, the dropsy in legs had eased, the speed of pneumonedema in chest was lowered and tumor sign had dropped from 140 to 128.

For a patient, family members' support is the best cure. Our son who lives with us had intended to learn abroad, but after his father was found to catch the disease, he decided to stay at home to accompany him. My husband is a pious Buddhist, but is unable to read aloud the scripture as usual after he got the disease. So our son does it for his father. As for me, in order to take care of my husband, I have resigned the teaching post in a middle school. Now the only wish of our family is for my husband to recover as soon as possible!

Change the ruthless prediction of death

Mr Yakeshima Nakashima jobless 64

I was lucky enough to know Tian Xian liquid in the anxious search for medicine

In July, 1998, the doctor told me that I suffered from lung cancer and could only live for "one year at the most and half a year at the least". I could not accept such fact and almost fainted then and there. I was at a loss and would like to try whatever kind of medicine that was said to be effective. So after reading the book entitled "Fighting against Cancer", I began to take Tian Xian liquid immediately 4 times a day at regular time plus Tian Xian pills.

Now although cancer has not disappeared completely, the tumor sign is lowering. Besides, my strength and mental status have recovered. Up till now, I have lived for one year and a half, more than what the doctor predicted. I myself felt it marvelous too. I believe I will recover health one day only if I continue with Tian Xian liquid. At last, I hope Mr. Wang will continue his research on medicine against cancer to save all cancer patients.

It was through newspapers that I got to know Tian Xian liquid and prolonged my life more than half a year.

175

A mother who goes towards the end of life with great courage

Taiwan Taipei jobless 76 Oral account daughter Lu Taitai

Grief over the loss of husband affected health

It has been for 4 years since mother passed away. Now, wherever I see old ladies with white hair, I will recall my mother as if she were with me. It was in 1994 that mother felt uncomfortable. At that time, I was hurt in an accident and mother and sister came to see me in San Francesco where I lived. Mother grieved over the death of my father, which seriously affected her health. Therefore, according to over 20 years' experiences in hospital, I felt that there was something wrong with my mother at the first sight of her.

Mother did not turned better after a period of time. So my elder brother took her back to Taipei. At that time, she coughed terribly, which might be caused by constant smoking, and could not fall asleep at night. Mother was eventually sent to hospital, but couldn't undergo further examination since she suffered from heart disease and diabetes. After several tests, the doctor said mother was likely to have lung cancer. But since she was over 70, the doctor could not suggest any effective treatment of western medicine.

I flew from San Francesco to Taipei as soon as I got permission from my doctor and fought against cancer with mother. I was the third of mother's 5 children. In childhood, I always felt that mother only paid attention to my sisters and brothers and neglected me. But the last period of mother's life was my unforgetable memory. I felt complete love from mother and was even envied by my brothers and sisters.

Enjoy a limited life to its full

Since the doctor declared giving up, my elder brother believed that traditional Chinese medicine was the only treatment for the disease and found Tian Xian liquid. Miracle occurred with the help of Tian Xian liquid and mother's will power to fight against cancer! Mother lived for another 17 months, surpassing the two months as the doctor had predicted!

During the 17 months, mother and I were either busy planning where to make purchase or flew to Hong Kong only to select a pearl necklace. Besides, I tried my best to arrange different people to accompany her to play mahjong, which is her favorite. There was no sign of "seriously ill patient" in the family. The only trouble was that mother could not sit on the chair for long, so brother found a massage expert who came to my home at fixed time to massage her. During the period I accompanied mother in hospital, I underwent gynecological examination and a tumor was found in my ovary. The doctor was not sure whether it was benign or malignant and told me it was safer to have it cut. But mother suggested me drinking 6 bottles of Tian Xian liquid like her.

In another examination one month and a half later, the doctor was surprised to tell me, "the tumor has disappeared, so it is not necessary to perform an operation." Therefore, Mother and I had more trust in the effects of Tian Xian liquid and never stopped drinking it afterwards. One year and a half later, mother was sent to hospital again maybe for her old age or for diabetes and heart disease.

There seemed nothing to be done except taking good care of her. Mother was not very clear about her disease. Four or five days before her death, she suddenly said that she wanted to eat fried chicken now and spareribs tomorrow. Seeing mother enjoying chicken so satisfied, my heart was bleeding, for I knew the last moment was coming.

Mother's finger nails, which were always painted red, seemed dry and thin in ordinary time. But on the last day, they appeared plump, tender and pretty out of a little dropsy. Doctors and relatives who visited mother unanimously appreciate her beautiful finger nails and toe nails. Mother was very happy, smiling, without knowing how sad we children were.

I told my brothers and sisters to be mentally prepared, not to let mother be inflicted, but to let her go through the last moment of her life calmly and peacefully. So we sign the agreement, giving up emergency treatment. Since I had worked in hospital for a long time, I was clear that the emergency treatment at the last moment was very cruel. On that night, when the electrocardiogram showed the parallel lines, mother stopped her breath and heart beat. I looked at mother peacefully without tears on my face.

Thanks to Tian Xian liquid, mother was able to prolong her life peacefully and I could have the most unforgetable 17 months in my life. Mother, calm without pain, set out another journey. Mother's face on that night will be branded in my mind forever.

It is not long before returning to society

Lim Mu Xin Fukuoka County private enterpriser owner 72

Six months left

In November, 1999, I was told to have suffer from lung cancer. The doctor repeatedly urged me to be in hospital, but I was too surprised to carry on normal thinking.

At that time, cancer cells had transferred to lymph in chest, so the doctor suggested treatment of traditional Chinese medicine instead of operation. This is how I got to know Tian Xian liquid. But after I took it for one month, the disease was not on the mend. Soon after the new millennium was celebrated, I was transferred to other hospitals for examination and the doctor was convinced that the tumor in the chest had developed into the fourth stage and had transferred to lymph node so that neither operation nor radiation treatment was possible. I was told to have six months' life left. Though I underwent the treatment of anti-cancer drug for 4 months, as had been planned, it was stopped for the side-effects.

Before the anti-cancer drug treatment, I found the dosage of Tian Xian series products instructed by the Japanese branch of International Cancer Recovery Association. I gave up the information obtained before and began to take Tian Xian liquid and Tian Xian pills according to the standard set by the Association. The trial this time did not affect routine dieting and on the other hand mitigated the side-effects.

In the first examination afterwards, the doctor said in an unbelievable tone, "generally speaking, the use of anti-cancer drug will not lead to so good effects." I was on the verge of telling him it was due to Tian Xian liquid, but I still enjoyed the improvement by myself. However, as the treatment became more frequent, the side-effects expanded too. Although suffering great pain, I was convinced that I was going to recover healthy and leave hospital. Before I was released from hospital, the doctor arranged CT and X-ray examination. X-rays showed that the primary cancer had reduced to undiscernible and cancer in lymph node also reduced in size.

When told that I took Tian Xian liquid and Tian Xian pills, the doctor said, "you are very lucky that the traditional Chinese medicine has produced such dramatic effects on this sort of cancer." I think anti-cancer drug alone was unlikely to so effective. So I'd like to express my sincere gratitude to Tian Xian liquid. Now I am resting at home and planning to return to work.

Although cancer cells have not totally disappeared in my body, it is not inappropriate to maintain the present the present state and exist with cancer. I will continue to take Tian Xian liquid in future and go to hospital regularly to prevent another attack or transfer.

I was once sentenced to having only six months left but have almost completely recovered now after treatment. I'd like to express my gratitude to the doctor who recommended me Tian Xian liquid and more to Tian Xian liquid itself.

"Hope" is always at the next turn

Mr Yamada   Chiba County   private enterprise owner   41

place all hope on the 80 percent effect

Many years ago, my husband had his thyroid gland cut for suffering from thyroid gland cancer. Nine years later, however, in April, 1992, the cancer transferred to lung, brain and neck. Since cancer cells spread to the two lungs, operation was impossible. The doctor told me directly, "there are at most 3 or 4 years left." In 1995, although strength recovered, his voice became hoarse; in February, 1996, blood appeared in phlegm.

When my husband was in hospital, I was considering other treatments and recalled books I had seen before about Tian Xian liquid. So I began to collect relevant information and have a deeper understanding about it. When I saw "over 80 percent effect", I rested all my hope on Tian Xian liquid.

My husband complained in disappointment, " even traditional Chinese medicine is no use now." I still did not give up a faint hope and encouraged him to take Tian Xian liquid 8 times a day. As a result, his physical state was improved and he was released from hospital.

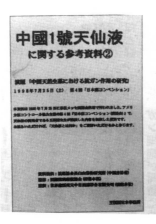
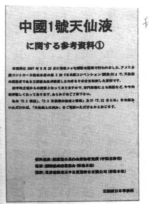

Never to give up easily

Lady Ishikawa Tokyo housewife 67

Unable to bear the violent side-effects

My wife was diagnosed as suffering from lung cancer in July, 1997 and operation could not be performed. Then followed treatment of anti-cancer drug and radiation. The doctor said that my wife could only live for 1 year.

After the fourth stage anti-cancer drug treatment in the early October, violent side-effects made her very weak, unable to stand anti-cancer drug. But cancer cells did not disappear completely with 20% left.

In late October, there showed sign of another attack, so radiation treatment continued. According to the examination in December, although cancer cells had not been eliminated completely, only a shadow was left. So my wife was released from hospital.

In May, 1998, lung cancer attacked again and transferred to brain. She was sent to hospital to undergo second stage treatment of anti-cancer drug and radiation on brain. It was finished in late June, but cancer cells remained in lung and brain. Considering my wife's physical state, the doctor said treatment could not be carried out any more. In other words, the doctor was powerless.

A miracle was achieved eventually!

I got to know the relevant information about Tian Xian liquid. After having a deeper understanding, I thought traditional Chinese medicine did no harm to body. So I bought it immediately. Since my wife used to suffer from pressure gastritis, I let her take two bottles of Tian Xian liquid per day from late May to make sure that it had no bad effect on stomach. In June, she began to drink 4 bottles per day. The examination in July showed that although cancer cells still existed in lung, those in brain disappeared.

Frankly speaking, Tian Xian liquid is not the only medicine we have tried. For my wife to recovery soon, we have tried almost all kinds of health food and medicine that may be effective against cancer, but with no effects.

In the short period of one month, cancer cells that even radiation could not kill were reduced in number. The effect is so dramatic! What we can do is only to say thanks.

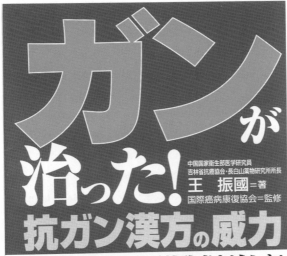

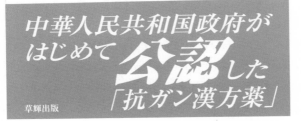

Iron-like will power

Chen Liangyi Taiwan Taipei veteran 60

An unacceptable blow

I always pay attention my health, for in the long term military service, an physical examination was arranged annually. I keep the habit after retirement.

In May, 1999, since I suffered from cold and cough for a long time, I went to hospital to undergo X-rays on my chest. The doctor told me that there was something abnormal so I had to be in hospital for further check. Eventually the doctor gave me a direct answer: you suffer from second stage lung cancer which is developing quickly. It is difficult to deal with it if an operation is not performed immediately.

I accepted the fact and faced the problem in the manner of a solder. Only if it can be tackled, I was not afraid. Different from other patients, it was I who comforted my wife and children. Then I underwent the operation and accepted the doctor's advice to receive chemical treatment after the operation. One third of the lobe of the lung was cut off , but the doctor was unable to eliminate cancer cells completely. So chemical treatment began immediately after the strength recovered.

During my stay in hospital to wait for the chemical treatment, my eldest son got information about Tian Xian liquid from his friends. It said that the medicine could mitigate the side-effects of chemical treatment, so my wife asked the son to buy it immediately. Besides, my son said his friend's mother also suffered from cancer. But since drinking Tian Xian liquid, no side-effects occurred during chemical treatment. But I thought my pension was only enough for daily expenses. The money for Tian Xian liquid would be a heavy burden to my son's family. Besides, I have served in the army for life. I could even sustain the pain for operation, let alone side-effects of chemical treatment. So I refused their kindness.

However, after chemical treatment the first time, I really felt uncomfortable, extremely tired and vomiting bile. I could not eat anything, even the food my wife cooked at home and took to hospital. I lay in bed with no strength to turn over. Regardless of my opposition my son called Hong Kong company to place an order for Tian Xian liquid and at the same time got the suggestions and points for attention from them. He told my wife to let me take the medicine regularly. Therefore, the side-effects of chemical treatment disappeared and I successfully finished the first course of chemical treatment which lasted 3 months.

I continue to take Tian Xian liquid up till now and go to hospital for further check regularly.

Now I take a walk every day and help my wife with housework. Sometimes I play Mahjong with my friends to exercise my brain. I think Tian Xian liquid does have some special effects. I believe as long as I take Tian Xian liquid regularly and pay attention to daily life to control the cancer cells remaining in my body, I can exist with cancer and lead a normal life. At such an old age, peaceful life is the happiest lot. I'd like to thank Tian Xian liquid for it has really helped me a lot. I tell it to other patients when I go to hospital for regular check. In a word, Tian Xian liquid is worth trying.

I can't be defeated for my family members

Lau Wai Hong Kong guard of a primary school 55

I took traditional Chinese medicine behind the doctor's back

I am addicted to sports, so I couldn't imagine my suffering from cancer. In September, 1996, I went to hospital for constant coughing. The examination showed that I caught lung cancer. Although I objected to an operation, I could do nothing under such circumstances.

Four months later, without detailed explanation of the condition of the disease, the doctor repeatedly carried out radiation and chemical treatment, which led to hair-dropping and weakening strength. But the doctor insisted on the above two kinds of treatment. At that time, my son happened to find information about Tian Xian liquid from internet and let me take it. I did not oppose traditional Chinese medicine. But the doctor in charge only believed in western medicine, so I had to take it behind his back.

After I began to take Tian Xian liquid, my physical state improved and hair grew again. In fact, the doctor already knew that I was drinking Tian Xian liquid, but what he learned made him unable to believe the effect of traditional Chinese medicine. He thought it was due to chemical and radiation treatment that my condition improved.

The combination of Chinese and western medicine must be the best cure

Since I began to use Tian Xian paste in June, 1998, dramatic effect has been achieved. Not only has the tumor in lung reduced in size, physical condition of the whole body has been improved a great deal. I can even resume work. Because of the pain remaining after the operation, I apply Tian Xian paste to relieve pain. As a result, I feel piercing pain only randomly. Later the doctor said that the tumor was brought under control and it was only necessary to have an examination once a month. So chemical treatment was stopped.

In order to maintain weight and health, I went to Tian Xian liquid agency not far away from my home to get a deeper understanding of dieting treatment. Generally, I'd like to try anything that might help cure the disease. At the same time, the responsibility of providing for the family and the sense of duty give me extra strength from inside.

I am lucky enough to be saved by Tian Xian liquid. I think Chinese people originally do not discriminate against traditional Chinese medicine. If it can be combined with western medicine, more lives can be saved.

Only when I fall ill do I realize that health is the heaven

Wang Zhouhong Malaysia owner of a shop 63

Operation can not be performed at old age

Considering public health institutions' repeated call for old people to have physical examination regularly in order to carry out treatment for disease at early stage, I went to hospital to undergo X-ray examination in March, 1997.

It showed a shadow in the left lung, which was diagnosed as lung cancer of 3cm x 2cm after further check. As the tumor was benign, it was only after more precise examination could it be decided whether an operation was necessary or not. However, due to my old age, the doctor finally decided on treatment with medicine.

In May, my son got the information from internet that Mr. Wang Zhengguo, expert on traditional Chinese medicine against cancer would make a diagnostic trip to Malaysia, treating patients free of charge. Thus, he got into contact with Mr.Wang via a friend. Mr. Wang immediately diagnosed it as lung cancer and instructed me to take Tian Xian liquid, Tian Xian pills and Tian Xian paste for one course of treatment (one month).

One month later, X-ray examination showed that the tumor was reduced to half the size. The effect was totally out of expectation.

In another examination on 25, October, the doctor told us that X-ray picture showed the tumor had disappeared completely. Hearing this news, I was overjoyed. It was with the help of Tian Xian liquid that I was able to escape from the trmendous pain.

Now although the tumor has disappeared, I continue to drink Tian Xian liquid at reduced dosage to prevent another attack. The recent medical examination showed "everything in normal condition". My appetite has recovered and I have become more energetic.

Re-enjoy the happiness of uttering sound from throat

Kan Mukkwun Hong Kong fire-fighter 54

Last April, I felt extremely tired and went to hospital for check. X-rays showed that I had lung cancer. The doctor said that an operation must be performed immediately. However, the pain in the lung did not disappear after the examination. In the doctor's opinion, it was because the operation affected rib. But seven months later, I could not even utter sound.

I was rushed to hospital and it was found that the tumor pressed vocal cords, which caused the loss of sound. In other words, cancer attacked again. The doctor could do nothing but give me some vitamins.

At that time, I remembered hearing of the effect of Tian Xian liquid and began to drink it immediately. In less than one month, my sound resumed. I went to hospital again and the doctor said that the tumor in lymph had disappeared and the sound in lung was no longer unclear. I was in good condition.

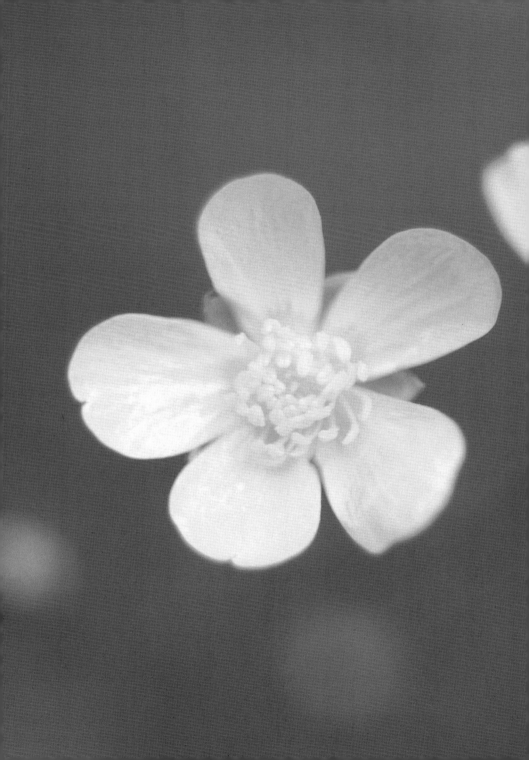

Experiences of defeating liver cancer successfully

Climb from the valley of despair

Mr Kido   Osaka   responsible personnel of a company 66

Place all hope on the newest radiation treatment

My liver does not function well for over 20 years and I take medicine given by doctor. I was diagnosed as suffering from C type hepatitis and received treatment of stimulant.

Two years later, data showed that the disease was brought under control and I was relieved. However, the disease deteriorated suddenly and had developed into cancer.

After I underwent liver artery embolism in July, 1998, I was almost cured. But cancer cells were found near portal vein. Another liver artery embolism did not achieve the same effect. It was like a bolt from the blue! In search of another treatments, I was told that hospital of Tokyo University was carrying out the latest "radio treatment", sending out radioactive waves from the top of needle through the wavelength of MICRO wave. It can once kill cancer cells 3 times more than before. So I immediately went to hospital of Tokyo University to receive that treatment.

However, that hospital is a research institute whose main function is not treating patients. Patients who covered a long distance to arrive here were transferred to other relevant hospitals on the grounds that there were not enough beds. I waited several months, only to be told that "your disease is beyond cure by any means" and made to leave.

At that time, the tumor invaded portal vein and transferred to three lymph glands. The lymph node swelled to 3 to 4 cm. Neither operation, nor radioactive wave or radiation worked!

"Is it really hopeless?" To my inquiry, the doctor in the digestion department answered coldly, " everyone is going to die, anyway. Although operation can still be performed, it's better to pray at home." And he added, "if you surely want to have a try, radiation treatment can be considered, but you do not have to be too optimistic."

Despair beyond description overwhelmed me and I could only glare at the doctor dumbfounded. That night, tears flowed the whole night and I could not close my eyes in the subsequent days and nights. Nurses kindly suggested me having a walk outside, "Be open-minded. Take a walk in Tokyo." Thus, my wife and I discarded all worry temporarily and enjoyed the happiness of shopping.

Hope emerged in darkness

Maybe the tour of Tokyo relieved me worry. I calmed down to consider what the doctor said. Finally, I decided to receive treatment in the radiation department of hospital of Tokyo University. Unexpectedly, doctors from different departments of the same hospital made quite different diagnoses, "Mr. Muhu, your disease is not very serious, so you do not have to worry about it." The new radiation treatment is controlled by a computer and only works on cancer cells. Besides, the side-effect is not so violent as before. What was even more exciting was that the doctor said there are hospitals of the same level in Guanxi area and they would transfer me there.

In November, 1999, I was sent to hospital to receive radiation treatment 25 times. In January, 2000, I underwent an embolism treatment for the newly found tumor in liver. It was at that time that I began to drink Tian Xian liquid, for I thought even if western medicine could cure the disease, the effect would not be most satisfactory if my immunity was not strong enough. So I placed all my hope on Tian Xian liquid. One month later, the tumors at portal vein, three lymph glands and liver were wiped out.

"How do they disappear?" When I asked the doctor, he said in surprise, "it is so incredible. I do not know what to say." Even the doctor could not believe the dramatic effect. A subsequent examination showed cancer of small size in the lung. The doctor said that radiation treatment could cure it, so I felt relieved. Although I got to know Tian Xian liquid only recently, I would continue with it in order to defeat cancer.

I was once thrown into great despair, but I am convinced that I am to climb from the bottom of valley one day.

How happy it is to live a peaceful life

Mr Kimura   Yamakuchi County jobless 59

I decided to fight against cancer till the last moment for my wife

It is over 10 years since cancer cells were found in liver. At that time, physical examination showed that my liver function was not good, so I was in hospital for further check. One year later, in 1989, on the day when Emperor Zhao He passed away, I was diagnosed as cirrhosis. Since operation was difficult for cirrhosis, I underwent liver artery embolism half a year later. In November that year, cancer was found in stomach. An operation followed to cut the stomach and gallbladder. At that time, my wife did not tell me the fact She hid the tremendous grief, actively took part in gatherings for cancer, read relevant information and bore all problems by herself. Two years later, my wife finally told the real condition to me. At that time, since I had ethanol injection treatment, a 12-cm-long cylinder must be inserted into my body. The pain was beyond description. What's more, much strength would be consumed. "How could you sustain such painful treatment if I did not tell you the fact?" My wife knew that it could not be hidden any more.

Frankly speaking, hearing the fact, I felt darkness before my eyes. How can I believe it? However, when I thought of my wife bearing so much pressure and pain for a long time, I decided not to demoralize. For my wife and family members, I must defeat cancer.

Going through the torture of long time treatment

From then on, I underwent ethanol injection treatment 20 times per year and from 1999 on was reduced to 9 times per year. My strength was consumed a lot after the painful treatment for a long time. but unbelievingly, I did not lose my appetite, so the recovery was quite satisfactory.

It was in April, 1999 that I got to know doctor Wang Zhengguo. My wife collected all kinds of news reports, magazines and books about cancer, in which she found Tian Xian liquid. Now, the tumor is 6 cm in size, neither growing nor reducing. Although it caused livery encephalitis last year, the disease cured by itself soon. And my appetite and sleep are no different from healthy people.

My wife says that almost all the other cancer patients we knew in hospital have died of another attack of cancer five years later. On the contrary, the doctor used to predict "impossibility of operation" and slight chance of cure, but now not only am I quite nimble in action, but keep a normal life. I have lived on for 10 years in this way and can't help feeling grateful. Cherishing the notion of "it must be cured", I keep on taking Tian Xian liquid.

During the period when I live with cancer, I enjoy life to heart's content, playing with radios, having a walk with the dog, growing vegetable, maintaining my interest and peaceful family life. Maybe the principle of "existing peacefully with cancer" can be really applied to the fighting against cancer.

Face disease with the will-power of climbing a mountain

Mr Horikuchi   Gunma County   employee of a company   70

Sustain the will power with the desire to climb a mountain

I originally suffered from C type hepatitis and received injection treatment in hospital once a week, but the disease had no influence on my daily life. I carried out work normally. In spare time, I liked taking photos of the beautiful scenery on mountains or engaged in gardening. Besides, I went to club to exercise the muscle to maintain the strength. Since I liked climbing mountain, I once tried mountain-climbing in winter.

However, last June, I felt slightly uncomfortable and went to hospital for examination. I was found to have liver cancer and the cancer cells had reached portal vein so that operation could not be performed. Even anti-cancer drug did not help much. Finally the doctor said that I could live for only three months. Slight as it was, there was still the last hope.

That was a new treatment developed by the medical institute of Jiu Liu Mi University, that is, inserting a duct from the inside part of thigh, injecting anti-cancer drug six hours a day.

With the wish to have a try, I told the doctor that I would undergo the treatment, "I'd like to accept whatever effective treatment. So please help me recover my health by means of modern medicine. At least, I could be able to climb mountain."

Break the prediction of three months' life

Since knowing my disease, my wife and I have read numerous relevant books. Whether medicine or health food, I've tried it as long as it is said to be effective against cancer.

Later we got to know Tian Xian liquid from newspaper. At first I was doubtful about it. But the more I understood it, the more I believed that I could be cured. My wife also encouraged me not to give up the hope of cure. So I began to take 3 or 4 bottles of Tian Xian liquid per day and 3 Tian Xian pill after each meal.

About one month later, the treatment was finished and I was released from hospital. The sign of recovery was even clearer. Afterwards, I received examination every two weeks and continued to take anti-cancer drug and of course Tian Xian liquid and Tian Xian pills. I, who had been sentenced to three months' life by the doctor, lived through the three months peacefully and celebrated the new year happily with family members.

But perhaps due to my old age, the resistance against disease and recovery was weakening. The aftereffect of the operation led to many inconveniences in my life and made me uncomfortable.

In January, 2000, I was sent to hospital for an operation to have the ducts pulled out and new ducts inserted. When radiography drug was injected into my body to show the state of liver, the doctor was surprised to say, "few people could have such a good recovery as you." Hearing the words when lying on the operating table, I believed it was attributed to Tian Xian liquid.

In February, ECHO examination did not find the trace of cancer. MRI and CT showed the same result. My excitement was beyond words.

Of course, it has not been made clear whether the combination of modern

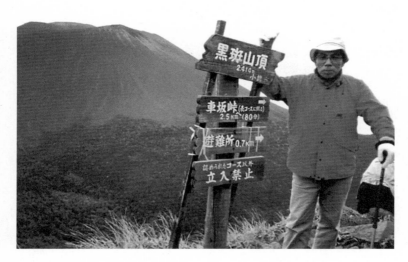

medicine and traditional Chinese medicine is absolutely correct, but I am sure it is due to Tian Xian liquid that I am able to defeat cancer. So if your family members, friends or acquaintances are inflicted by cancer, please recommend Tian Xian liquid to him or her, for hope and beautiful future lies here.

Never to admit failure

Lady Sawada   Byogo County housewife   77

Take in strength in daily activities

I underwent an operation for breast cancer 10 years ago and afterwards had regular examination twice a year. In the summer of 1997, cancer was found in liver. Another operation was performed immediately and ethanol injection treatment was carried out twice together with anti-cancer drug. Due to the violent side-effects of anti-cancer drug, I lost my appetite and couldn't take in food for nearly 3 months. Thus, treatment had to be stopped. At that time, a relative introduced Tian Xian liquid to me.

I had thought that "all medicines taste terrible". But it is not so in fact. Tian Xian liquid is not so difficult to drink at all. At first, I took 2 bottles every day. Later on, in the hope of quick effect, I drank 6 bottles of the liquid per day. As I expected, radiation examination showed that the shadow in liver disappeared and blood test proved the same surprising result.

Then I received injection of anti-cancer drug twice per month. Since I drank Tian Xian liquid every day, no side-effects occurred and I could enjoy the delicious food. During the later period of staying in hospital, my good appetite and sleep even surprised the nurse. Now I drink 4 bottles of Tian Xian liquid per day to prevent another attack and continue with it in future.

I am impetuous in nature. I am not worried after catching the disease, nor do I keep myself busy in order to forget it. I put all the housework to the responsibility of my son and my daughter-in-law. I spend every day as usual.

Thank Tian Xian liquid for helping me return to life, relieved of the worry for the disease, enjoying the happiness in the family and the simple and normal life.

If asked how I was able to defeat the monster of disease, I think "not admitting failure" is the secret of fighting against cancer.

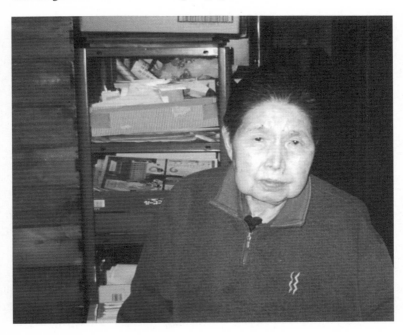

Trembling with the only wish for recovery

Mr Shimada   Kanagawa County   employee of a company 65

Negligence led to disaster

I have the build of an athlete, enjoying playing baseball and taking pride in my strength. But after 50 years old, the function of my heart weakened and returned to normal after treatment.

In Autumn of 1998, my bowel was not regular and even with blood. Afterwards, my strength was weakening and my mood was even worse.

In February next year, I was found to have rectum cancer and underwent an operation. The doctor suggested vaccine. Unfortunately, personnel transfer in the hospital delayed the injection of the vaccine to one month later.

One week after the injection of vaccine, the doctor told me that the cancer cells had transferred to lung and liver. So an operation was to be performed on my lung and anti-cancer drug was to be injected into my liver. I had expected not to suffer the pain of operation any more, but in face of the disease, I had to bestir myself to receive treatment courageously. At that time, my son sent Tian Xian liquid, Tian Xian pills and relevant information. So I began to take it.

Two weeks later, I was permitted to go back home. However, I caught diarrhea and vomiting out of negligence and had to return to hospital. Since I felt flatulence in my belly, drip feeding was injected into my body. Thus, in order to defeat cancer, I decided to pay more attention to minute details, for if I continued to be so careless, the recovery would not last long.

The treatment on liver began shortly afterwards. A duct was inserted into the liver and anti-cancer drug was injected into the liver through the duct. Out of my expectation, the side-effect was rather slight. I only felt somewhat tired and sleepy, slightly hot all my body and a little sour in my mouth. I believed it should be attributed to Tian Xian liquid and Maruyama vaccine. And Tian Xian liquid played an even more important role, for I felt energetic soon after I drank it. A operation on lung followed one month later. X-ray check before the operation showed two tumors of different sizes in the left lung. But in the operation, only the bigger one was found and cut away while the smaller one disappeared. I was more convinced that it was eliminated by Tian Xian liquid and Maruyama vacine.

Then, after another injection of anti-cancer drug into the liver, the treatment which lasted 100 days was finally finished. From I was released from hospital up till now, I continue to receive the injection of anti-cancer drug every two weeks and to take two bottles of Tian Xian liquid and six Tian Xian pills per day and Maruyama vaccine every other day.

The doctor once told my wife, "there is no hope for your husband. You shouldn't take it to heart too much." But now, not only has my weight recovered to that before the operation, I can even do simple sports like walking, climbing mountains and playing golf as well as carry out some light work in the office. I am trying to return to my normal life.

My quick recovery is not only owed to my wife and all the relatives and good friends but also to doctor Wang Zhengguo, inventor of Tian Xian liquid. Thank you!

Never to let father die of cancer

Mr Oishi   Kanagawa County   owner of a private enterprise   64

The whole family were thrown in great sorrow

On the morning of October, 2, 1999, my father suddenly felt very uncomfortable and vomited a basin of blood! He was immediately rushed to hospital and was found to have stomach cancer, which had transferred to liver and developed into the fourth stage. There was only one year's life left! After the whole stomach was cut away, it was found that the tumor in the centre of liver had grown to 7 cm and the two small tumors at the two sides 2 cm, which could not be cut away.

It seemed as if the whole family were thrown into the bottom of deep

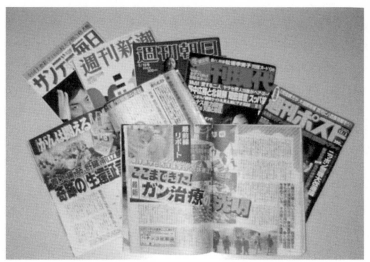

valley. Our mind was totally blank with the only obsession that we can't let father die of cancer. In search of good treatment, the advertisements in newspapers, which I had no interest in before, caught my eye. In order not to let slip any chance, I got books about Tian Xian liquid according to the advertisement. After reading it carefully, my confidence in Tian Xian liquid enhanced.

After the operation on stomach, father was in high fever for the whole week. Not only was the appetite lost, the weight also dropped 10 kg. When the fever was lowered, I suggested father drinking Tian Xian liquid. In doubt, father began to drink 6 bottles of Tian Xian liquid every day. As a result, not only did excretion turn better, he grew more vigorous gradually. So father continued to take it regularly per day.

It was originally planned that father would take anti-cancer drug after strength recovered. However, in time of the coming new year, father was released for hospital temporarily. During this period of time, father did not take any other medicine except Tian Xian liquid. Unexpectedly, father's complexion became more ruddy and strength was obviously recovering.

Later on, due to the side-effects of anti-cancer drug, he was afraid of being weakened and thus lying on bed all time. At that time, a friend told us that a kind of treatment that anti-cancer drug could be injected into liver directly without much side-effect and the patient could even go to work normally. So we transferred to another hospital and underwent the treatment up till now. Besides, drip feeding injection and Tian Xian liquid are also continued.

It is one year since father was found to have the disease. Although he has lost almost 20kg, cancer cells did not transfer after operation and father could maintain a normal life. All this is attributed to Tian Xian liquid.

I can not retrospect the time when I was lying in bed with disease

Lady Hirashima Hiroshima County   employee of a company 53

I wrongly thought of myself as fully recovered

Two years ago, a polyp was found in large intestine in a physical examination and an operation followed to have it cut. I did not take a small polyp seriously and as I was leaving hospital, the doctor said, "the malignant part has been cut away. So you do not have to worry. To be cautious, take 3 anti-cancer pills per day. If there appears nothing wrong in the following two years, it means you are fully recovered." So I was even more relieved. And the first examination after I left hospital did not show anything abnormal, so I thought I had fully recovered.

One year after the operation, it was found unexpectedly that cancer cells had transferred to parts including liver. I was too amazed to say anything. When I underwent radiation treatment, I really felt if I kept on ignoring it, I would lose my life one day!

It happened that my daughter bought a book written by doctor Wang and visited me in hospital. I read each paragraph and each chapter carefully. After leaving hospital, I began to drink Tian Xian liquid. The regular examination afterwards did not show anything abnormal. In other words, I was very health. So I returned to work.

Now, I took Tian Xian liquid 6 times a week. No matter how busy I am, I never forget to put 3 bottles of it in the pocket of my uniform praying that Tian

Xian liquid "helps improve my immunity". Besides, I drink a big cup of juice mixing root-tuber of aromatic turmeric (granule), citric acid, carrot, banana, milk and sesame.

Not only my life was saved, but my mind

Now, both my excretion and appetite are normal. My strength and mental state are satisfactory. The preceding two years are branded in my mind. When I was in hospital, I once asked a nurse, "can I return to normal life after the treatment is finished?" Her answer was, "once cancer has transferred, most of the patients will be sent to hospital again."

I did not expected the nurse to say something so cruel to the nervous patient in such a light tone. I was filled with anger, "by no means will I live in hospital again and see that nurse!"

At that time, I couldn't fall asleep either before or after the examination. When family members talked about Spring Festival or Pure Brightness, I was obsessed with the thought whether I was able to live till that time. Hearing others say some piercing words, I couldn't help losing my temper. I spent every day in bad mood.

Frankly speaking, Tian Xian liquid not only saved my life but also my mind. My gratitude to Tian Xian liquid is beyond words.

I believe, so I recover

Putlapun Thailand owner of a private enterprise 53

The only trouble now is that I am over-weight

In June, 1998, a tumor of 9cm x 10cm was found in liver. The diagnosis was cancer at late stage and the doctor said there was only 6 months left. After being treated with anti-cancer drug twice, I was tortured by side-effects like vomiting, hair-dropping and felt pain in the affected part constantly, though the tumor reduced in size.

In November, my friend introduced Tian Xian liquid to me, so I began to drink 60ml per day together Tian Xian pills and Tian Xian paste. Soon, the pain and other symptoms of my body were mitigated.

Three months later, all symptoms, including jaundice disappeared. An examination in February, 1999 showed that the tumor reduced to 8.2cm x 8.3cm. Although the doctor suggested an operation at that time, I refused, for I believed Tian Xian liquid could cure my disease. I continue to take Tian Xian liquid and Tian Xian pills up till now.

As a result, the tumor was growing smaller and smaller. In May, 2000, it reduced to 6cm x 7cm.

It has been 2 years since the doctor sentenced me to 6 months' life. My life and work are no different from that before. Later, the doctor who once suggested an operation also said, "since the tumor is reducing, an operation does not seem to be necessary." When my weight increased from 75kg to 93kg, the doctor even reminded to stop growing fatter. So the only trouble now is to avoid being over-weight.

Wife's great care gets back my health

Puttawala Thailand 52

It started from a traffic accident

Ten years ago, in a traffic accident, I had my rib broken and liver and spleen seriously hurt. Since I originally had a B type hepatitis, it developed into cirrhosis. At the beginning of this year, the disease began to deteriorate. The flatulence in belly, ?水, fever and tiredness tortured me.

The examination in hospital found tumors in liver and bladder, which were diagnosed as cancer. However, the doctor neither told me the fact nor made instructions of treatment, but only asked me to "receive check regularly".

At that time, how lucky was I to know Tian Xian liquid through friends! I was quite suspicious about the effect at first. With an idea to have a try, I began to take 60ml of Tian Xian liquid and 12 Tian Xian pills per day.

Since my physique is featured as "internal heat", I had a fever and dropsy about my eyes as I began to drink it. The agent doctor for Tian Xian liquid told me, "the present symptoms show the sign of recovery. It could be mitigated by drinking more water." He asked me not to worry and continue to drink it.

Dramatic change

One month later, not only the above symptoms, but also flatulence in belly, water accumulation?水, fever and tiredness that had troubled me for long all disappeared. The dramatic change enhanced my confidence in Tian Xian liquid and my reliance on it.

Half a year later, all the discomfort kept away from me, and I became more vigorous physically and mentally. I could even drive my beloved family members to have a trip. What is more exciting to me is that the latest examination showed that "all cancer cells disappeared".

I continue to drink Tian Xian liquid to prevent re-attack. However, my recovery is owed more to my wife who takes great care of me than medicine, food and sport. She makes the schedule for my taking medicine, doing sport, diet. Without the support and care of family members and, the most important, Tian Xian liquid, I could not have recovered so quickly.

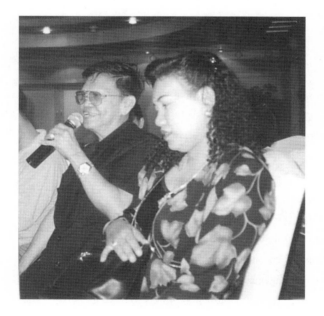

Never to give up!

Mr Nakaro Miyagi County Owner of a private enterprise 49

Chemical treatment did not take much effect

In April, 1998, my 49-year-old brother underwent an operation on large intestine cancer (sigmoid flexure). After the operation, he began to drink 500ml juice decocted from 5 gram Sheng Yong after he was able to take in water.

Urine returned to normal after a period of time and the side-effect was not very serious. The recovery could be called successful. He mainly ate vegetables, replaced meat with fish and continued to drink Sheng Yong juice.

About ten months later, it was found that cancer cells had transferred to liver. The doctor suggested an operation or one of the two chemical treatments. My brother decided on the direct injection of anti-cancer drug once a month, three times a course. But tumor sign did not change much during this period.

Convinced that the disease can be cured

In November, 1999, radiation treatment was conducted as soon as it was known. At that time, I encouraged my brother and sister-in-law to read the book entitled "Fighting against Cancer" and take Tian Xian liquid as soon as possible. Thus, from December, he began to drink 4 to 6 bottles of Tian Xian liquid and continued for half a year. Since my brother does his work outside, he often feels thirsty. However, since drinking Tian Xian liquid, he feels quite smooth in throat.

In June this year, I had a chance to go to Hong Kong and, with the help of the Japanese branch, visited the headquarters there. Under the instruction of the headquarters, my brother began to use Tian Xian paste as well. He himself often said that Tian Xian paste really made his digestive system unobstructed. Afterwards, he received the treatment of induct insertion, as was planned, to cure the remaining tumor.

Now, my brother still takes Tian Xian liquid together with 2 Tian Xian pastes according to his physical state.

Although there is the sign of recovery, the it is still not the most desirable result. But we are sure that the disease can be cured with the efforts of my brother and those around him.

It is like a nightmare when I look back

Mr Oshima   Chiba County   jobless   62

Complex double cancers

In February, 1997, I was diagnosed as suffering from bile duct cancer at the anus and rectum cancer at the upper part. Shortly afterwards, I underwent catheter treatment on 3 parts. But operation couldn't be performed on bile duct cancer and chemical treatment took no effect at all.

The doctor said that only radiation treatment could be tried. Thus, in January next year, I was transferred to another hospital that could carry out radiation treatment. An operation was performed on rectum cancer in April. In May, catheter treatment was stopped and I was released from hospital. However, in less than two weeks, cancer attacked me again and I was sent to hospital to undergo catheter treatment again.

From then on, I began to drink Tian Xian liquid occasionally. I first knew Tian Xian liquid from the books and information sent by my friend. I was quite doubtful about it. In July, 1998, doctor Wang Zhengguo came to Japan to make a speech. My family member went to listen and recorded his speech. After I listened to it carefully, I decided to bet my life on Tian Xian liquid and drank it seriously.

Formerly, the doctor had told me, "the cancer transferred to liver is incurable, for the cancer cells cause ascites. So the possibility of cure is rather slight." I said to myself, "if I do not go back home nos. Maybe I can't go back …" So I left hospital.

However, in the second month after I began to drink Tian Xian liquid seriously, not only did jaundice lower, ascites also disappeared. Catheter treatment was stopped in the fourth month.

Now, small tumor still exists in my body. However, recalling my frequent visits to hospital for cholangitis and weakening function of liver, it is really like a dream.

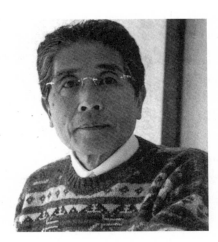

It is better to live even one day more

Mr Ikeda   Saidama County   employee of a company   51

Searching for traditional Chinese medicine suitable for me

My husband's liver is always not in good condition and he goes to hospital for treatment. One day, my husband's physical state seemed quite abnormal, so I suggested him having an examination in hospital. It showed that the cancer had developed into late stage. The doctor said that there was at least 2 or 3 months left. The unbelievable fact made me tremble. Darkness pervaded before my eyes.

When my husband left hospital two months later, he, who had no idea of the reality, was very distrustful and uneasy. Family members tried to make life return to normal and relieve him of pressure. No matter what happens, we tried our best to restrain ourselves. I vowed to help him live on! However, gradually my husband seemed to have guessed his disease and began the search for suitable traditional Chinese medicine. Thus he came to know Tian Xian liquid and began to take it.

Tian Xian liquid does differ from other traditional Chinese medicines. Shortly after he began to drink it, his mental state kept improving day by day. I couldn't suppress my happiness. Recently, my husband seems even more energetic than us. It is five years since he was sentenced to several months' life. He continues the physical examination regularly now. The tumor has been very small.

Benefiting a lot from Tian Xian liquid, my husband suggested Tian Xian liquid whenever family members or friends fall ill. Now my energetic husband works even better for his beloved family members.

Curb the horse at the cliff, and get back health

Mr Oda Tokyo jobless 69

Stopping taking medicine recklessly led to another attack

In October, 1988, the medical examination at hospital showed that cirrhosis had developed into liver cancer of 1cm x 2cm. Thus, I underwent liver artery embolism and ethanol injection, etc., which did take effect.

The condition lasted two or three years and then I saw reports about Tian Xian liquid from magazines. I immediately collected more information and read it carefully. Then I began to take it.

At first, I drank 4 bottles of Tian Xian liquid per day. It took effect quickly. The supersonic wave examination showed that the shadow of cancer disappeared. So I reduced the amount of Tian Xian liquid to two bottles per day.

In the examination in November, 1997, a tumor of 1.2cm was found again. So I again drank 4 bottles of Tian Xian liquid every day.

The examination in October, next year showed that the tumor did not increase in size, nor deteriorated. Now it can be deemed that I have recovered.

Finally I can enjoy a peaceful life at an old age

Lady Namiki   Kanagawa County   housewife 78

Cancer has not attacked again for three years up till now

In the ECHO examination in November, 1995, a shadow was found at liver. Next January, it was confirmed to be a liver cancer of 4cm x 4cm. I was sent to hospital in February. An operation was impossible due to my old age, so I had to receive embolism treatment.

However, it did not take any effect, so I left hospital. In April that year, I knew of Tian Xian liquid from magazines. After I got a deeper understanding, I began to drink 4 bottles of Tian Xian liquid one week before I went to hospital in June.

I underwent embolism treatment again in June. Two weeks later, my appetite recovered and my complexion became ruddy. One month later, the examination showed that the tumor reduced greatly in size, which surprised the doctor.

Although the doctor suggested continuing embolism treatment, I refused on the grounds of my old age. I continued drinking Tian Xian liquid only. After months later, in January, 1996, the examination showed that the tumor had disappeared completely. The tumor sign was only 1 digit!

In fact, as my physical state was recovering, I stopped drinking Tian Xian liquid for the following two years. As a result, the cancer attacked again. Now I am undergoing embolism treatment, and at the same time, drinking Tian Xian liquid. in fact, for a patient who suffers from both cirrhosis and liver cancer, re-attack is most likely. I think I'd better drink at least two bottles of

Tian Xian liquid for the sake of prevention.

Now cancer has not attacked again for three years so far. It can be deemed that I have recovered completely. I am sure it is Tian Xian liquid that takes effect.

The nightmare that keeps worsening finally stops

Mr Tokokawa   Kanagawa County   jobless   67

Operation again and again

I am not very strong. It is not only easy for me to catch cold, but I am bedridden for two or three days every time I fall ill. I am accompanied by medicine for cold, and have constipation occasionally.

The physical examination in the summer of 1994 showed that I suffered from C type hepatitis, which developed into cirrhosis soon. At the beginning of next year, in the operation to have my spleen cut away, tumor was found in part of the liver. So I underwent ethanol injection treatment, but the effect was not so good as expected.

In 1996, the tumor grew bigger and bigger, so I had to have one third of my liver and gallbladder cut away. In 1997, it developed into livercancer. Up till now, I have received five liver artery embolism operations.

It was after the second operation that I began to drink Tian Xian liquid. Thanks to Tian Xian liquid, my strength recovered soon and appetite has become as good as before. More important, it curbs the deterioration of the tumor.

Slip from the crevice between fingers of the god of death

Lady Efuji   Byogo County housewife 51

Twelve years ago, I had the breast cancer removed. Three years later it transferred to uterus and I had to have my uterus cut, too. Cancer cells till existed in my body and transferred to lung another three years later! The doctor said that if the tumor was not removed, the cancer cells would spread throughout the whole body. So I underwent the third operation.

Afterwards, I went to hospital once a week for regular examination and receive the treatment of anti-cancer drug. But it did not take effect. After a period of time, I became very tired, either mentally or physically, and lost my appetite. The CT examination in the designated hospital showed there was a cancer of 3 cm in the liver.

The doctor said that even the continuous treatment for liver cancer couldn't prolong one's life much. So my family members sought advice from the doctor on traditional Chinese medicine for cancer and accepted the suggestion of Tian Xian liquid. At that time, I knew nothing about traditional Chinese medicine. Urged by my family members, I began to drink Tian Xian liquid.

I remember clearly that it was November, 16, 1997. Two weeks later, I did not feel tired any more and my appetite recovered.

At the beginning of next year, I continued to drink 20ml of Tian Xian liquid and went to hospital every two weeks for regular examination. In middle of October, it showed that the liver cancer reduced from 3 cm to 1 cm and blood returned to normal too. The doctor was also surprised at my quick

221

Inspire the determination to fight against cancer

Mr Cheng Chi Keung   Hong Kong   jobless 67

Bear tremendous sufferings only for survival

Nearly one year ago, I suddenly felt itching on my hands and feet. So I went to Ma Jia Lie hospital for check, but the doctor only informed my wife of the result. Afterwards, I found my wife somewhat strange. With my repeated inquiries, she finally told me the fact.

"Perhaps it is liver cancer. The tumor is so big that the operation can't be performed. The doctor said that there is at most half a year left. Radiation and chemical treatment may prolong the life two years if it is successful."

It was so unacceptable like a bolt from the blue. I had to undergo the treatment of anti-cancer drug and radiation for the two years' life. But it only added to my sufferings.

Maybe it was due to luck that I got to know Tian Xian liquid from my wife's friend. My wife and daughter told me not to worry about money, but to grasp each chance of cure. I thought that even if it led to economic burden, it would only last half a year. In order not to disappoint my wife and daughter, I began to drink Tian Xian liquid.

Unexpectedly, an miracle was achieved. My physical state improved! My appetite came back and sense of flatulence disappeared. Insomnia, which was caused by dysphoria and itching and was inflicting me disappeared. I could have a sound sleep till next morning.

Thus, I make up my mind to fight against cancer. I stop taking anti-cancer drug but only rely on one bottle of Tian Xian liquid per day. I believe as long as my physical state is recovering, it can generate enough strength to defeat cancer. Although I still feel slight itching on my skin, I feel calm and energetic.

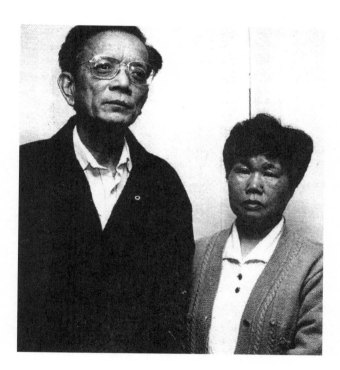

Feel the beauty of life

Jun Wan Taiwan Taipei writer 58

I was once weary of life for the violent side-effect

During the past 12 years, cancer has attacked me three times, breast cancer, uterus cancer first and then liver cancer two years ago. Physical sufferings and great fear made feel that life was so weak.

To what degree were the most advanced examination techniques, operations and chemical treatment of modern medicine able to control my disease? But the side-effects of the treatment were so unbearable sometimes that I even did not want to live on! One of my father's friends, who is a doctor of traditional Chinese medicine, instructed me how to combine western medicine and traditional Chinese medicine, which displayed great function in the treatment for cancer. With the help of my father and that doctor, I began to take the traditional Chinese anti-cancer medicine "Tian Xian liquid", which is developed by means of modern technology.

Tian Xian liquid not only relieved me of the suffering from side-effects caused by western medicine, such as vomiting, difficulty in swallowing, hair-dropping. Besides, my strength improved and hope to live arose. The doctor in charge and friends were surprised at my robust life. Tian Xian liquid really helps me defeat cancer.

Anyway, I'd like to thank the doctors and nurses who tried their best to save me. It is with their help and support that I am able to see light in darkness once again and pick up writing.

Recalling my struggle against cancer, I feel as if I were a leaf of grass braving the strong wind courageously, never receding in face of the hardships and growing robustly in the warm sunshine. Life to me is not only important but also more beautiful.

Now I do not live only for survival. I'd like to encourage all patients to go through difficulty.

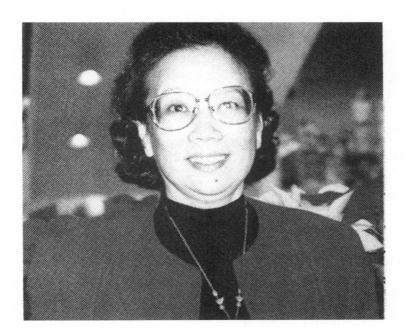

Health returns to me

Chen Wumei   Taiwan Taipei housewife 70

There was still no sign of improvement with all treatments

"Mum, you are likely to have liver cancer, but the doctor said that you are sure to recover as long as you receive treatment in hospital. Don't worry. Let's pray together···"

When my son told me the fact, I was not too much surprised, but only felt a little sorry. My youngest son is in charge of Zhi Yuan Jing temple of Taipei Buddhist Association. So every morning I go there to pray and have acquired a sort of understanding.

In fact, I lost appetite and felt extremely tired for some time. And my belly swelled until internal haemorrhage occurred. I was sent to hospital immediately.

Later my son told me that the doctor's diagnosis was "liver cancer at late stage". Besides operation, all the other chemical treatments did not take effect. I was still in a dangerous state.

The disease underwent a drastic drastic change in one year

Thus, I became a frequent visitor of hospital for half a year. Since my son has some communication with the Nai Liang Temple Japan, someone of them, after knowing my disease, told us that "there is an anti-cancer traditional Chinese medicine called Tian Xian liquid from China and it can be bought in Hong Kong. Seeing me getting weaker day by day, my son went to Hong

Kong in person.

Since my cancer was at the late stage, I drank eight bottles of Tian Xian liquid every day and continued for half a year. The examination half a year later showed that cancer cells disappeared! I got fully recovered in only one year.

Five years have passed. Not only have I recovered my appetite, but I no long suffer from insomnia and pain in my joints which has tortured me for a long time; health has returned to me.

Besides, my weight dropped to 45kg before the operation and to 38kg after it, but now is 52 kg. My son begins to worry again, "mum, you are too fat ..."

227

I am not lonely on the way of fighting against cancer

Mr. Dong Taiwan Taipei teacher 56

I can't remember how many years ago in blood donation, I was told to carry B type hepatitis virus. From then on, I began to be careful of my daily life, including diet. I never drink and go to bed at fixed time. Even my family members are weary of such life, but I insist on it, for I know B type hepatitis virus will likely develop into serious liver disease.

In April, 1999, all the four people in many family were infected by the flu spreading the whole town and went to hospital to take some medicine. However, when my wife and two sons recovered, I still felt tired every day and lost appetite as if the food I ate got stuck in stomach. I thought it was due to maldigestion or medicine for cold that I felt so weak. On one night, I suddenly felt a piercing pain in the right upper abdomen, which made unable to sleep. I got up to find pain-killing medicine in the drawer, ate two pills. Then I felt somewhat better and fell asleep.

I thought it was neuralgia, for I did not feel the pain in the following two days. But on the third day, as I was giving lessons in school as usual, a fit of great pain made me bend my waist. The students saw me turn pale in a cold sweat all over and sent me to clinic in the school. The nurse arranged to send to hospital immediately and informed my wife to go there. The doctor inquired me about the condition in recent years and told me that I would undergo several medical examinations. Finally he asked me to take it easy in hospital.

In waiting for the examination, I did not need my wife to accompany me in hospital for I could go around by myself. When I felt well, I walked around happened to visit me after school. The sight gave them a surprise, for they had never seen their father and mother so intimate since they had knowledge of the world. However, when they saw the grave expression on our faces, they asked anxiously what had happened. I tried my best to calm down and told them that their father had liver cancer and was waiting for treatment now. My big son blurted out that his classmate's father lived in the next ward and also suffered from liver cancer. Besides treatment in hospital, he also took a traditional Chinese medicine. I thought he must be referring to the patient I chatted with the day before yesterday.

My big son immediately went to ask his classmate's father for the materials about Tian Xian liquid. My wife and I began to study it carefully, skipping the part we did not understand and discussing with each other. We waited for the doctor's decision to see if Tian Xian liquid should be taken too.

The next day, the doctor said that since the tumor was so close to the main vessel that operation was difficult to perform. So he decided to carry out embolism treatment first, which had slight side-effect, and then supplementary treatment according to the result. At that time, I was able to give sober consideration to the condition. I saw free call in the materials and tried dialing the number. Out of my expectation, it reached the home office of the company in Hong Kong. The lady who answer the phone explained in detail their service. What attempted me to have a try was that the lady said that when you asked about our products, you should let us know your condition and the treatment you underwent at the same time, so that we could know how to help you.

I felt that the company was very objective, so I took the medicine according to the instructions of the lady. I also asked the patient next door in the ward and, in chatting with family members of the patient in the bed beside me, I was told that the patient suffered from liver cancer at the late stage. I felt it very strange why they put me in such a ward. The following day, I went to the neighbouring ward to find someone to chat with and saw a patient read some materials in bed. I took one book randomly. It was entitled "A Good Cure for Cancer: China No.1 Tian Xian liquid". Seeing him in high spirits, I began to chat with him.

He told me that he suffered from liver cancer at the fourth stage. With the recommendation of his friend, he had drunk Tian Xian liquid for 3 weeks, so that he was able to read some materials by himself. Besides, he said were it not for Tian Xian liquid, he would have already died.

I felt a little sad and began to think: Does the doctor also suspect me to have liver cancer so that he put me here? When my wife visited me, I told my doubts to her. Before I finished, tears came into her eyes. She gazed at me and said that as soon as I was sent to hospital, the doctor knew from the supersonic waves that there were two tumors in my liver, one of 7.5cm x 8cm, the other of 3.5cm x 1.5cm. The further check was to see where there was still chance of operation or other treatment.

It was a hard blow to me! I was dumbfounded! I did not know what would happen to. Would I be reduced to skeleton with a big abdomen like the one next door? My wife's tears seemed to have dried up. I wouldn't accept such fate! I was only 56. Why did cancer attack me, who led such a regular and normal life? I wanted to shout, but couldn't make any sound. I was also afraid that shouting aloud would break the tumors in the liver.

Face in face with my wife, suddenly she threw herself into my arms. We hugged each other, hoping that time could stop! At this moment, my sons about the condition after taking the medicine. Thus, the so called combination of western and Chinese treatments was carried out.

I left hospital ten days after the embolism treatment was finished. I continued to drink Tian Xian liquid and often contact the office in Hong Kong for consultation through the free call. They also instruct me on matters that deserve attention in daily life and dieting. I feel that they are not only selling medicine but taking care of every patient in the real sense. I maintain contact with my son's classmate's father. He shares the same feeling that we are being taken care of by a group of people who are really concerned about patients.

My wife also calls Hong Kong for matters of attention on dieting and can always get satisfactory answers and instructions. Now I pay more attention to my physical state and ask my whole family to take care if themselves and dieting. I do not want that another one gets affected or my sons can not be taken good care of after I, the backbone of the family lay down.

I have been drinking Tian Xian liquid for over one year and pay attention to daily life. My family are even more closely knitted! I want nothing but more time I can spend with my family members. Tian Xian liquid really helps a lot and the company is guiding me.

Also, I'd like to thank all people in China-Japan Fei Da Company for their assistance. I would more value what I have now! I am not lonely on the way of fighting against cancer, for I get great support. Although it is a big expense, I believe life is much more important than money.

I'd like to pay any cost only if I can live one day more!

Re-enjoy the love between grandparents and grandsons

Mr Nick Mark   U.S.A New York business consultant 62

It was a pity that the cancer was not detected earlier

I suffered from diabetes before 40 and tried various medicines, but the liver function kept deteriorating. When the medical examination showed the bad condition of the liver and suggested further check, the doctor in charge of diabetes said that it was likely to anyone. So I give up further check. But the condition kept worsening. In early June, 1992, after I was transferred to another hospital, I was found to have C type hepatitis and sent to hospital immediately to have stimulant injected into my body. Maybe it was due to the medicine, this time I did not remain in hospital for long.

The next year, after having a trip with the whole family, I found blood in my stool. The diagnosis was large intestine cancer. The operation cut off a part of 1.5cm from the large intestine. The doctor felt regretful that "it is a pity that the cancer was not detected earlier". Afterwards, I returned to work for one year but was physically weak. At home, I could do nothing but lying. Soon I was sent to hospital again for liver cancer. After chemical treatment for some time, I received an operation which lasted over 10 hours. The doctor told me that large intestine cancer had transferred.

Recovered strength and re-enjoy the happiness of life

After the operation, I suffered from the pneumonedema in abdomen, and I took diuretic to get rid of it, but protein was lost too, so protein was complemented through drip feeding.

Unexpectedly, the doctor said my lymph gland might have been hurt and therefore I had to undergo another operation. Although the operation showed the lymph was in normal condition, there appeared white power in the liver. So it was certain the cancer had transferred. The doctor declared I could live for only several months. At that time, I got to know Tian Xian liquid from news report and began to drink 6 bottles of it every day immediately. Several days later, bits and bits of white power appeared in the ducts connected to me.

When I asked the doctor about the white power, he avoided a direct answer, but only said, " you can go home if you want." I thought I was going to die. Maybe the doctor himself did not know what the white power was.

However, it may be due to Tian Xian liquid, the pneumonedemain abdomen began to reduce, so I underwent an operation to have the pneumonedema reduced. About one month after the operation, the ducts connected to me were all taken away and I was released from hospital. Now my strength has recovered and I can take care of my beloved plants as before and send my grandson to school and meet him when school is over. All this is given by Tian Xian liquid.

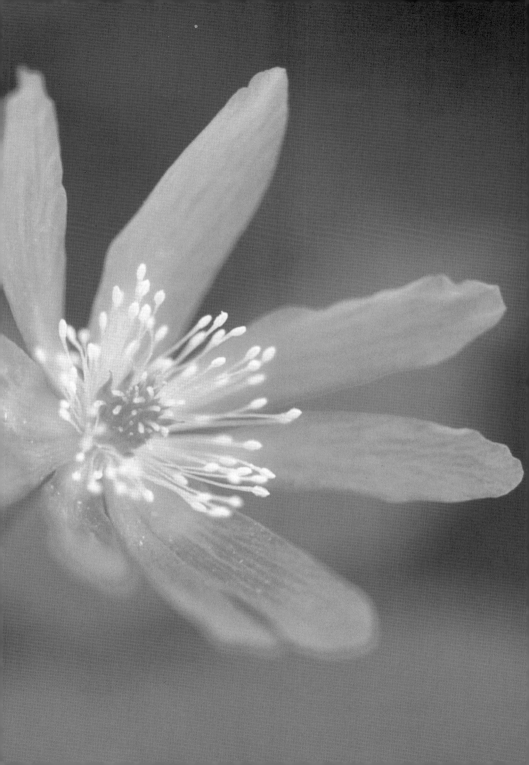

Experiences of defeating stomach cancer successfully

Make good use of medicine and regain life

Mr Obune Tokyo employee of a company 55

In August, 1997, I was diagnosed as suffering from stomach cancer, which was progressive. An operation followed immediately. Two years later, it transferred to the lymph glands about the artery in abdomen and the doctor said that I could live for only one year.

I decided to defeat cancer and began to take Tian Xian liquid and anti-cancer drug. As a result, three months later, the tumor reduced in size. At the end of March, this year, it reduced quickly and my wish was going to be realized. But I suffered a lot from the side-effect of anti-cancer drug. In the state of uneasiness, I felt settled to take immunity-improving and anti-cancer traditional Chinese medicine Tian Xian liquid. Seeing my present condition, few would believed that the doctor once predicted that I could live only half a year, or at most one year.

In the middle of August, after the third examination, the doctor in charge confirmed again that the tumor kept reducing. In fact, I was expecting that cancer cells might have been wiped out thoroughly, but on the other hand, I reminded me sensibly to keep alert, "how could it be so east?", for CT showed that cancer cells still existed, as if grasping me. Anyway, I myself was surprised at the quick recovery in a year.

In face of the monster of disease, keeping a good mental state plays a significant role. Long time treatment is sure to lead to mental tiredness. Besides, the disease is on the mend at one time but deteriorating at another. So it is necessary to keep us in good mood. Both the mental and physical conditions should be taken into consideration. The doctor once predicted that I could live only half a year, or at most one year but I have survived peacefully for over one year. This is the most important. Now I declare aloud that I can "take a breath". I had prepared "declaration of returning to life", but since tumor still remains in body, I can only say "take a breath".

Like all the other patients, I have gone through various ordeals and thought a lot. So I made a web page of my experiences of fighting against cancer in the year, in hope of providing a place for patients and their family members to think. The web page is the result of my explorations, with my blood and energy woven into it. Entitled "how to defeat cancer", it not only records the treatment in hospital but also illustrates how I struggled for chances of survival as well as my personal experiences in defeating cancer, which, I hope, could be shared with other patients who have suffered from cancer. If my experiences could be a reference for defeating cancer, it will be a greatest honor to me.

It is a very serious and important issue to fight against cancer, so I hope that every one of you can provide some information, advice, feelings, problems, etc. for exchange and discussion. Now I wake up at 5 o'clock and have a walk near my home. Today I met the couple I have communicated for many years. We haven't met for two years and it really seems a long time. We greeted each other and seeing them in deep love and healthy, I felt myself in a good mood, and thought that I should make even more efforts. I hope all the other patients will never give up and continue fighting like me!

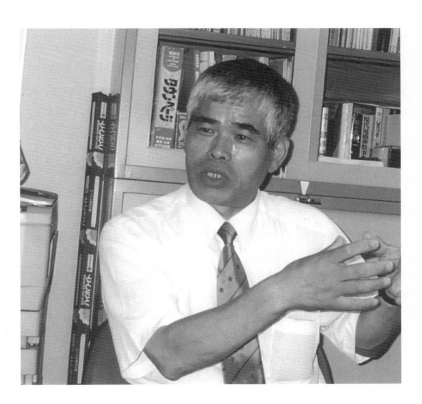

Start from the victory of Wei Qi competition

Mr Furotaka Tochigi County jobless 74

In march, 1999, the doctor diagnosed me as suffering from stomach cancer and cut off two thirds of the stomach. Although I recovered, my physical state kept worsening from June, 1998, with my weight dropping and strength weakening. "Does cancer attack again? Or does it transfer?" the ill omen was haunting me. Then, I went to hospital for examination once a month and regular blood test. Soon, the cancer indicator (CAI 9-9) was little higher. The normal range is 35-37, but mine was 118-125, 153-180 and was climbing month by month and even reached 248 in December, 1998.

At that time, I saw books written by doctor Wang Zhengguo and began to drink Tian Xian liquid immediately.

After the examination in January, 1999, the doctor in charge collected all my family members and told them that the disease attacked again, hoping that they were mentally prepared. However, after drinking Tian Xian liquid, it was so marvelous that my strength was recovering. Nine months later, I took part in the Wei Qi competition organized by the local government out of interest and became the winner! To win in a limited period of time, it is important to concentrate attention. And to bring what is achieved in training into full play, mental and physical strength is necessary. If one is in bad physical state, it is difficult to win. As for me, I really feel my strength recovered in the competition.

In January, 2000, I went to hospital for various examinations. In the ECHO examination conducted first, the doctor said that it was no different from last time. After the CT on abdomen, endoscopy, X-ray examination on chest were done one after another, the doctor uttered the result that made me happy, "everything is normal." As the doctor in charge expressed satisfaction with the result, I thought that it was all due to Tian Xian liquid.

For the seven years, the so called treatment is nothing taking medicine and examination which invariably shows "nothing wrong". So I am convinced that I should thank the mysterious power from medicinal herbs in Chang Bai Mountain that helps me defeat cancer.

The one who survives cancer is standing in front of me

Mr Kobayashi Kanagawa County jobless 71

In the autumn of 1998, I was found to have progressive stomach cancer in the annual health examination. However, the endoscopy did not showed anything wrong and I did not feel uncomfortable. After I accepted the doctor's

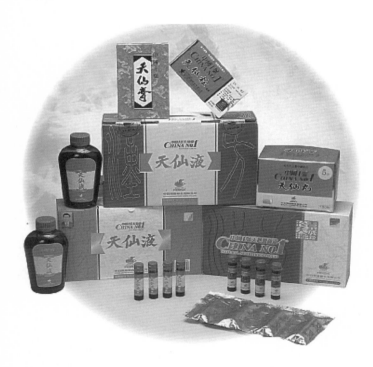

advice of operation, I began to collect information about cancer. I had no idea of cancer and I should thank my relatives and friends who collected for me relevant information, which brought Tian Xian liquid.

When I contact the Japanese branch of International Recovery Association, the consultant told me a case of a female patient. She suffered from ovary cancer, but, after taking Tian Xian liquid and Tian Xian pills, recovered much to the doctor's surprise. So a gained much confidence and fought more courageously against cancer.

Recalling the patient's courage and with friends' support, I was convinced that "defeating cancer only depends on Tian Xian liquid", so I began to drink it before the operation.

The operation finished successful. Two weeks later, I began to drink Tian Xian liquid again and then undergo the treatment of anti-cancer drug. Thanks to Tian Xian liquid, I was relieved of the side-effect and finished the treatment. All people were surprised and delighted. I was even more convinced of the effect of Tian Xian liquid.

From I was released from hospital to now, I have continued to take 4 bottles of Tian Xian liquid and 4 Tian Xian pills. Up till now, the regular examination half a year shows that everything is in normal condition.

However, since the whole stomach was cut off, I became weak temporarily, but recovered well. Now both my mental and physical state is good. I can help my wife do some cleaning, shopping, washing, etc. and am happy to read and arrange the yard. My friends say that I do not look like a patient at all.

In order to prevent transfer and defeat cancer, I decide to continue drinking Tian Xian liquid. I, who was once faced with death, values every day of life so as not to let me regret.

Go out of the shadow of anti-cancer drug

Lady Takada Shiga County housewife 58

It was at the end of 1998 that I knew mother suffered from stomach cancer. It was so unexpected that mother, who was always so energetic no matter what disease she caught, was found to have cancer in the health examination which was intended for prevention. It showed that mother's stomach cancer had developed into the third stage and the doctor declared that mother could live only one year. We did not tell the real fact to mother, but only told her that it was ulcer and an operation had to be performed to cut off three fourths of the stomach and the surrounding lymph glands.

Although the doctor suggested an operation, I was still sure that there were other medicines that could prolong her life besides western medical treatment. As I was in search of the medicine, my friend introduced Tian Xian liquid to me. Without delay, I let mother drink it one week before the operation.

After the operation, since mother was still not told the real condition, she did not drink Tian Xian liquid half a year. However, when the cancer cells transferred to the pelvis, we had to tell mother the truth. Mother decided to rely on Tian Xian liquid and began to drink it again.

Soon, cancer cells transferred to ovary so mother had to have the two ovaries cut off. When receiving intravenous injection of anti-cancer drug regularly, she not only maintained strength but recovered quickly, which surprised the doctor in charge, for generally the side-effect of anti-cancer drug would cause the weakening of immunity and strength. But mother can still carry out housework lightly and even do not lose appetite. Both mother and all family members thank Tian Xian liquid. I think it would be another situation if we only relied on western treatment.

Up till now, mother continues to drink 4 bottles of Tian Xian liquid every day. The doctor once predicted that mother could live only one year, but she lives up till now with the help of Tian Xian liquid. Of course, it does not mean that there is no likelihood of another attack in the future, but my mother and I will make efforts together.

"Believe it" is the best treatment

Mr Nosaki Tokyo Company Director 65

On June, 7th, 1999 when I was undergoing regular health examination, the doctor found something wrong about my organ and suggested further check. The unexpected terrible news was like a bolt from the blue.

The next day, I took the X-ray photo that showed something wrong and went to the hospital attached to K university to visit professor G, who is surgeon. He diagnosed it as "progressive stomach cancer" and suggested that operation to remove the cancer be the best treatment. I thought to defeat the disease, a close relationship must be established between the doctor and the patient, so I decided to undergo the operation.

Although I could not imagine who powerful cancer is, I knew it was increasing per second in my body. The result was unimaginable if nothing was done quickly to stop it.

Besides, I also chose to drink Tian Xian liquid after having a deep understanding of it. Traditional Chinese medicine is different from western medicine that produces a dramatic effect on certain symptoms, but emphasizes the improvement of physique and reduction of side-effect.

I thought if the doctor said that anti-cancer treatment was necessary, I should drink Tian Xian liquid beforehand to mitigate the side-effect. Or some dramatic effect would occur or maybe the tumor was found to be reducing in size so that operation was unnecessary. They were all possible, weren't they? If so, I might as well drink it 4 times a day.

As I was in hospital, I put forward the idea of drinking Tian Xian liquid to the doctor in charge and got his permission. So I continued to drink it till the night before the operation. So all together I drank Tian Xian liquid for 22 days. I had hoped that in the examination before the operation, I could be told by the doctor that the tumor disappeared or reduced. In fact I was very disappointed.

But I still believed that Tian Xian liquid could more or less prevent the growth of the tumor and assist the successful completion of the operation. The doctor said that the lymph test after operation showed that cancer cells did not transfer to the 55 lymph nodes that had been cut off and blood test also did not show any trace of transfer. He said, " the result is even better than expected."

I took it for granted that since the tumor had been removed, cancer cells disappeared. I really did not want anything unexpected for I had paid such a cost.

Now I know it is not due to the successful operation that cancer cells did not transfer. I believed it should be attributed to Tian Xian liquid, which fought against the cancer cells in my body.

After the operation, I walked around to quicken the heal of the wound and, after I could take liquid food, I ate liquid food five times a day to maintain the function of my digestive organ. It was not easy, for, besides avoiding eating too much, which would lead to reverse flow, I had to pay attention not to eat indigestible food, which would cause serious result if the food obstruct the digestive organ. As I was about to leave the hospital, the nutrition doctor told me repeatedly to follow the principle of what to eat and what not, but I did not expect it so difficult to abide by.

I was released from hospital three weeks after the operation and resumed drinking Tian Xian liquid four times a day. It exerted great pressure to drink it at fixed time, but the time was calculated according to the physiological response. To defeat cancer, I should stick to the schedule.

Drinking Tian Xian liquid, I felt a sense of comfort from the bottom of my heart. It is very important to choose the most suitable one from the various anti-cancer medicines in market, believe it and take it under instructions. The

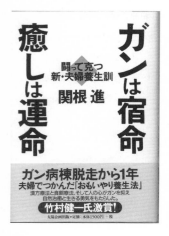

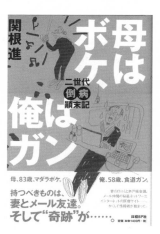

kind of Tian Xian liquid I drink is "Strong China No.1 Tian Xian liquid". Some patients feel it difficult to drink. As for me, maybe I am a little obtuse; I neither taste its flavor nor felt that I am taking medicine, but some nutritious liquid. In a word, I do not react violently against it.

After I was released from hospital, I knew a book entitled "Mother is stupid and I suffer from cancer" (written by Guan Gen Jin and published by Ri Jing BB Publishing House). Most people may have read the book, which accounts one's fighting against esophagus cancer in the form of diary. It is quite meaningful to cancer patients and their family members. Tian Xian liquid is also mentioned in it.

During the author's stay in hospital for esophagus cancer, he obtained much information about cancer from the internet, relatives and friends, and finally chose SOD advocated by Dr. Tu Zuo Qing Shui Dan Yu and Tian Xian liquid by doctor Wang Zhengguo. As he received treatment in hospital, he also took the above two medicines. As a result, the tumor reduced in size and finally disappeared. So he refused the operation and returned home well.

Recently, Mr. Guan Gen published the sequel "cancer is the fate and recovery is the destiny" (Sun Planning Publishing House). The book not only gave a detailed introduction of Tian Xian liquid, but also described the author's visit to the research institute of doctor Wang Zhengguo in Chang Bai mountain. We are moved by his action and feel his courage in face of cancer by reading the book. For patients who drink Tian Xian liquid, Mr. Guan Gen greatly inspires them. It is 1 year since the operation and there is no sign of transfer or another attack. Six months ago, I reduced the amount to two times a day in order to prevent transfer or another attack. I sincerely hope that I can recover successfully and keep away from cancer.

Feel the essence of life again

Mr Watase Saga County employee 56

In May, 1999, I was found to have a type of progressive stomach cancer and underwent an operation immediately in Social Insurance hospital in He Zuo county. About three fourths of the stomach was cut off and I stayed in hospital for a week.

At that time, my daughter, who was in Tokyo, came back to He Zuo to take good care of me and bring a gook about Tian Xian liquid. Before I finished reading the book, I was eager to drink it as soon as possible.

One week after the operation, I began to drink Tian Xian liquid with the doctor's permission, 10ml every four hours and 6 times per day. The doctor had said after the operation, patients would feel suppression in the chest and sometimes vomiting without exception, so I did not have to worry. But not once did I vomit, so I recovered successfully.

After the operation, I received the injection of immunity medicine for a week but did not feel any side-effect. I thought it must be due to Tian Xian liquid. However, my weight dropped from 80kg to 65kg after the operation, but rose to 75 kg 1 year later and to 80 kg 3 years later. My stomach also recovered to normal condition and so did my appetite. Even the doctor was surprised. The doctor in charge once said that the cancer might attack again in two years. However, 3 years have passed and there is no sign of attack. The examination every three months did not show anything wrong either. Now, my life has returned to normal and I also return to the fire fighting post and begin to do sports.

My sincere suggestions

Lady Kishima Tokyo housewife 79

My mother passed away eight months after the operation. Nevertheless, I still want to write down my feelings to provide some reference for those hopeless patients.

When my mother was diagnosed as having stomach cancer, it had transferred to large intestine and pancreas. The operation cut off the whole stomach and a large part of the pancreas and large intestine. In other words, all parts with tumors had been taken out.

After the operation, mother began to drink Tian Xian liquid with aunt's introduction. One month later, the nurse who took care of my mother asked curiously, " are you taking something that could provide nutrition for the whole body?" It is obvious that mother recovered quickly and so she was released from hospital. We all thought that it was attributed to Tian Xian liquid, so mother continued drinking it at home. As a result, the side-effect of anti-cancer drug did not occur.

However, the examination in the third month after mother left hospital showed that the cancer indicator rose a lot. The doctor suggested taking concentrated anti-cancer drugs, which was the last way out. Although the violent side-effect was paralleled before, the effect is over 60%. Should we accept the suggestion or not? All the family members were troubled by the choice, and finally decided to receive the treatment. About one month, mother began to vomit terribly and suffered from serious stomatitis, so that she was unable to drink Tian Xian any more.

Why did not we let mother drink Tian Xian liquid non-stop? We feel greatly regretful now! Although mother began to drink Tian Xian liquid immediately after leaving hospital, however, it was too late. She was sent to hospital again. This time she was unable to return home. Later, we came to know that when Tian Xian liquid could not be drunk, it could be replaced by Tian Xian suppository. Although we could not confirm the anti-cancer function of Tian Xian liquid in mother's case, it was absolutely true that her strength recovered after drinking it. Mother's case can show that Tian Xian liquid is sure to help mitigate the side-effect of anti-cancer drug of low density. However, when mother received the treatment of concentrated high density anti-cancer drug, side-effect was unavoidable. The shelves in bookstores are lined with book about the experiences of "miracles of defeating cancer", which mention shark cartilage, water soluble KITOSAN, vitamin treatment, AGALIKS young pilose antler, loquant leaf warm pressure treatment, etc. We had tried all available and tried Tian Xian liquid at last, which proved to be the most effective traditional Chinese medicine. Unfortunately, miracle was not achieved on mother. But I still believe Tian Xian liquid is the only one that may create miracle.

I believe in miracle

Chen Wenchao Taiwan Gaoxiong veteran 60

For a long I felt pain in stomach whenever I ate food and I always felt uncomfortable, either vomiting or hiccuping. In June, 1998, I was diagnosed as suffering from stomach cancer and underwent an operation immediately to have the whole stomach cut off. Only after I recovered strength gradually did my wife tell me that the doctor said before the operation that, " the cancer keeps deteriorating and has transferred to the whole body. So life is threatened." So it was necessary to have the whole stomach cut off. Only then did I know that I had lost my stomach.

Since I am pessimistic in nature, I slightly felt that I might have caught stomach cancer before I was told the fact. So it was not a great surprise to me. I was released from hospital the next month. My wife got to know Tian Xian liquid from magazines and read the relevant books carefully. When she saw that Tian Xian liquid is particularly effective against stomach cancer, she bought it immediately and let me drink it at the beginning of August.

My family members reiterated that "it is absolutely effective against cancer" and with the recovering of my strength, I felt myself the real experience of "absolutely effective against cancer".

All the friends and relatives who have visited me are excited to see that I am on the mend. I am convinced that the miracle is created by Tian Xian liquid. I will continue to drink Tian Xian liquid to defeat cancer completely, for I am sure that I will recover health one day.

253

Cancer disappears in my body

Yeung Ching Wan   Hong Kong   housewife   58

It has been nine years since cancer was found in my body. At that time, I was doing cleaning work in a bank. One day I fainted and was sent to hospital. the endoscopy showed there was a polyp in my stomach, which was confirmed to be cancer.

The doctor said, "when first detected, the tumor was small like a bean. It was suspected to be gastritis. However, the tumor grew rapidly. In one month's time, it was in the size of an egg. If it continues to transfer at such speed, even an operation is difficult. The patient could only live for two or three weeks!" The unexpected terrible news amazed all the family members, but they pretended to be calm in order not to let me sense it. However their manners aroused my suspicion that I might catch some incurable disease.

I did not want to die out of no reason and asked the doctor directly. Showing me the X-ray photo, he told me that "I could only live about one month." I was too surprised to anything. I left hospital without operation or other treatment. I last wish was to go to the end of life with the company of my family members.

At that time, a relative of mine told me that " my mother had her lung cancer cured after drinking Tian Xian liquid. You'd better have a try." I accepted his suggestion and began to drink Tian Xian liquid, thinking "I could at least relax myself a bit if life can be prolonged". Out of expectation, I stopped vomiting and recovered my appetite. Subsequently, after drinking Tian Xian liquid for a year, the egg-sized cancer in stomach was found to have reduced to that of a bean. Another examination showed that cancer cells had disappeared completely.

Treatments selected for patients at an old age

Lady Kurosawa Hokaido housewife 87

I still remember that it was in November, 1995, mother said that she always felt sleepy after getting up. "I feel as if I am going to faint if I stand up immediately." Gastroscopy showed that stomach cancer attached again (CEA 2.7). Due to her old age, the doctor gave up medicines of violent side-effect, but prescribed some traditional Chinese medicine. However, the effect was not so good as expected.

Thus, in February next year, my eldest brother who worked in Taiwan took back Tian Xian liquid, an anti-cancer medicine which is said to be quite welcome there. So mother began to drink 4 bottles of Tian Xian liquid per day. To our delighted surprise, CEA dropped to 2.0 in March and to 1.6 in May. It was on the decline. In August, we took it for granted that mother had fully recovered, so she stopped drinking Tian Xian liquid. Consequently, in the middle of October, she was infected with acute enteritis with a fever above 40 degrees and diarrhea which lasted three days, so she was sent to hospital and was released about one month later. But she had a diarrhea again and CEA rose to 2.7.

Later, in January, 1997. She began to drink three bottles of Tian Xian liquid again till October when CEA dropped to 1.4 and kept under control. Then she reduced the amount to 1 bottle per day.

Now, mother does not feel pain at all. Although she is still physically weak, her digestive function is quite good and she says she can taste the delicious food.

Mother is of old age; she has a bad memory and can't fall sound asleep. But for me, these are the most luxurious troubles.

Choice as to accepting silently or changing life

Lady Noda Tokyo housewife 64

About ten years ago, I was busy working in Mother Ballet Classroom and nursery and my big daughter was in hospital. Maybe the overwork broke me down. Finally the acute pain and feeling of vomiting drove me to hospital. The doctor thought it necessary for me to stay in hospital for further observation on the grounds of stomach disease. The unexpected change surprised me. In my life I was hospitalized only for the operation on caecum and for giving birth to children. But now I had to stay in hospital.

After I underwent various checks, an operation was performed to cut off the whole stomach. I was released form hospital two months later but was sent there again and doctor injected drip feeding into my body. Without knowing what had happened, I felt there must be something wrong. At that time, I felt terrible sick, all the hair dropped and I even had difficulty in taking in food.

Since I had no knowledge of medicine, only after my husband told me, did I know that the doctor let me take anti-cancer drug to prevent transfer. In a work, the side-effect of anti-cancer drug made me suffer terribly so that I was unable to think seriously. After leaving hospital, I was weakened by the operation on stomach. In order to avoid obstruction in intestine and reverse flow of food, I had to eat very slowly, otherwise I could not swallow the food.

Thus ten years have passed. My husband and I still have trips to other places, and I also have energy to take care of my grandson. Life is no different from before. As I was going to relax myself, the physical examination showed something wrong about my digestive organ and needed large intestine endoscopy. I think many people have undergone such examination. Before that you should not eat food to let the large intestine empty and clean and drink 2 liters intestine cleaning water. In my present condition, I have to drink a small of nutrition at two times, let alone 2 liters intestine cleaning water. So I had to give up the examination. One week later, I went to hospital to receive intestinal lavage and blood test and the doctor suggested further observation.

My husband, who underwent the operation on stomach cancer like three years ago said, "you'd better drink Tian Xian liquid with me." But it was so difficult to swallow. At that time, I got to know that "natural nutritious liquid" was added to Tian Xian series products, so I began to drink it immediately. Unexpectedly, it is so easy to drink. Every day I drink two bottles of it smoothly.

Although natural nutritious liquid is different from Tian Xian liquid intended to kill cancer and has the same function as other nutritious liquids, yet it still can help improve immunity and is beneficial to health for it contains the same medicinal herbs as Tian Xian liquid. After drinking it for one week or ten days, I have found that such symptoms like daze or breathlessness are mitigated and I no longer feel cold in hands and feet but warm all over myself.

Although I have to continue to undergo regular blood test, I expect a lot from "Natural Nutritious liquid".

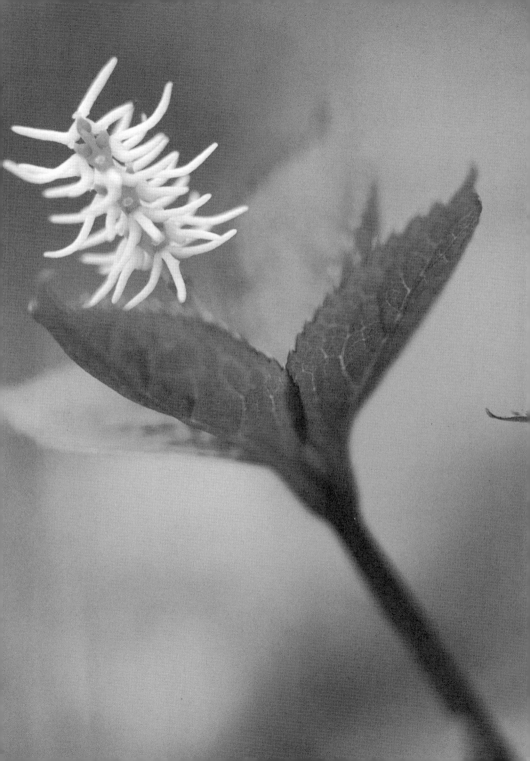

Experiences in defeating intestine cancer successfully

Find stronger life in cancer

Lady Okubo Kanagawa County housewife 67

As a proverb says, "find a floating wood when drowned in water", in June, 1996, after medical examination in three hospitals, the doctor showed me the X-ray photo and explained, "sigmoid flexure cancer, the fourth stage". It flashed through my mind, "how could it be possible!" But I could do nothing but listen to the doctor silently. After I stayed in hospital for a week, I thought it was time for the operation. The doctor told me to wait for a time.

Subsequently, the doctor in charge explained to us that "there is some small shadow in the lung and it is better cut off it together to avoid another operation". Another doctor told us that "you should endure the great pain after the operation". My husband and I could say nothing.

The operation lasted five hours and I was released from hospital two weeks later. At that time, I was surprised to see books and advertisements about "defeating cancer", saying that doctor Wang Zhengguo would deliver a speech during his visit to here. I decided to listen to his speech to have a deeper understanding. Doctor Wang's instructions at the speech were easy to understand, so I began to drink Tian Xian liquid after I understood it fully.

The effect was so marvelous. The medical examination did not find anything wrong. Now I swim every day to keep healthy and continue to drink

Tian Xian liquid until I get fully recovered.

I should thank my husband for letting me know Tian Xian liquid. He lived in Man Zhou from 13 to 19 years old and during the following 50 years established good relationship with China as a member of China-Japan Friendship Association. At first, I did not really trust traditional Chinese medicine. I was so lucky that my husband applied for the participation of the speech for me. Now, although medicine in Japan is advancing quickly, ideal treatment after operation has not been developed. Most cancer patients have to explore better treatment by exchanging mutual feelings. As a result, those who do not want to tell others their disease or want to talk about it or want to know others' condition are isolated and live every day of their life by themselves. For them, the Japanese branch of International Cancer Recovery Association is the best source of information. Not only can you know the result of various treatments and the process of developing a new medicine, but you can also know other patients' feelings and experiences. I hope that other patients suffering from cancer can go out of the shadow into the sun as soon as possible.

Defeat cancer with absolute confidence

Mr Odachi Miyagaki County owner of a private enterprise 48

On December, 9, 1999, the doctor diagnosed my husband as having progressive rectum cancer. An operation which lasted four and a half hours was performed the next day. Seeing my husband sent to concentrated treatment ward with many ducts inserted in his body, I couldn't help crying.

Accompanied by my daughter, I carefully listened to the doctor in charge explain the slice of the tumor taken out. Although the cancer cells did not transfer, the tumor was exposed from the rectum and extended to the lymph-vessels around. The visible part of the tumor was wholly taken out. It was like a swollen 九孔. Sitting in the doctor's office, everything was so vague before my eyes as if they had nothing to do with me.

Although I couldn't accept the fact, I was at loss and still had to appear energetic to cope with customers. However, when I returned home, I couldn't help crying. "Cancer equals death", the notion was haunting all the time. I have such a good husband. Why is the God so unfair to me?

The day before my husband was released from hospital, the doctor in charge told him about the rectum cancer, operation and the plan for taking anti-cancer drug. Although he said firmly, " I will try my best to cooperate the treatment", I could still feel his surprise.

Afterwards, among the information about cancer I collected, I found Tian Xian liquid developed by doctor Wang Zhengguo. With the assistance of the Japanese branch of International Cancer Recovery Association, we came into contact with people mentioned in the book. From then on, I was convinced that only Tian Xian liquid could cure my husband.

Subsequently, my husband began to take anti-cancer drug for five days per month, which lasted six months. At the same time, he also drank Tian Xian liquid. The combination of western medicine and Chinese medicine avoided any side-effect, which greatly surprised the doctor. Several days ago, my husband underwent a detailed examination seven months after the operation and it showed that the newly generated cells at the suture were quite normal.

When I recall the time when my husband was found to have cancer, I feel a lot. Now the whole of my family vow to "defeat cancer" and we believe that only if he continues to drink Tian Xian liquid, cancer won't attack again. Thank Tian Xian liquid.

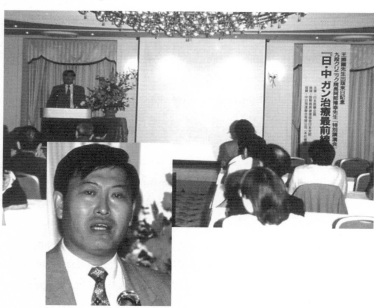

A miraculous extension from 6 months to 2 years

Mr. Huang   Gaoxiong Taiwan   housewife 57

It was in 1997 that mother was found to have rectum cancer. She went to the provincial hospital for check for she suffered from serious diarrhea and was unable to take in food.

The doctor said that the cancer had deteriorated terribly and an operation had to be performed immediately to cut off the whole rectum. He also told us that mother could live for six months only. Mother was not told the real fact.

Some time after mother stayed in hospital, a friend introduced Tian Xian liquid to us. Since it was known through the sister of the doctor in charge, we had thought it was the medicine from the hospital and let mother drink it.

Since relatives and friends introduced numerous kinds of medicine, we treated Tian Xian liquid just as an ordinary medicine. Unexpectedly, the medicine took particular effect. When mother's strength recovered to a degree, she was released from hospital. Soon, she was on the mend and returned to her normal life.

When flu spread at the beginning of this year, mother caught flu. Then cancer cells were found to have transferred to many parts, including peritonaeum, which led to intestinal obstruction. Mother was unable to take in food at that time.

Every day, I prayed the god to create a miracle as soon as I opened my eyes. Western medicine could not help. We let mother drink Tian Xian liquid to prolong the life. Unfortunately, she still left us one month ago. Tian Xian liquid is the only medicine mother took after leaving hospital, which prolonged her life up till now.

The half a year's life that the doctor declared was finally prolonged to two years. During this period of time, my sister and I accompanied mother day and night to enrich her life at the last moment. We should thank Tian Xian liquid and I think mother, who is now in heaven shares the same opinion.

Reliance of body and heart after operation

Chen Yueyun Malaysia jobless 37

In October, 1999, the doctor diagnosed that there was a tumor (third stage) at the bottom of large intestine (sigmoid flexure). She underwent an operation in the cancer specialized hospital and had artificial anal opening installed. After the operation, the doctor suggested radiation treatment. My sister happened to have worked in the Malaysia Agency of Tian Xian liquid, so she was clear that if the radiation and anti-cancer drug treatment was complemented by Tian Xian liquid, the result would be better.

She also has a thorough understanding of the side-effect of anti-cancer drug and radiation treatment. So the whole family gathered together to discuss whether to receive the treatment.

Finally, we decided to give up radiation treatment and relied on Tian Xian liquid only. So three months after the operation, she began to drink Tian Xian liquid and, after another months, added Tian Xian pills up till now. My sister did not receive any other special treatment, but she has good complexion and is recovering her weight. The examination in hospital showed that cancer cells disappeared. We are all excited! Thank Tian Xian liquid for putting my sister's disease under control.

From sharing happiness to experiencing in person

Mr Kawada Hiroshima jobless 61

In February, 1995, the sudden melena greatly surprised me and the family members agreed to send me to hospital immediately for a check. The diagnosis was rectum cancer and I underwent an operation immediately. Fortunately, the operation was very successful and about one month later, I was released from hospital.

I continued to take the medicine given by the hospital and suffered a lot from its side-effect. Six months later, my niece who used to have uterus cancer recommended Tian Xian liquid, a traditional Chinese medicine to me for she recovered by drinking it. So I began to drink Tian Xian liquid. As a result, I got fully recovered half a year.

Five years have passed and the two physical examinations per year do not show anything wrong. I return to normal life. Now I still drink Tian Xian liquid and after the condition becomes stable, I often have trips domestic and abroad. Now I am in good physical state and even more energetic than before. The happiness of recovering health is beyond words.

I continue to drink Tian Xian liquid although the amount has been reduced greatly. I think it a good way to keep healthy.

Family members give me the courage to struggle for survival

Mr Fred Walltic U.S.A. driver 52

At the beginning, I felt myself weakening, the weight dropped sharply and finally I was even unable to drive the bus. After the examination in a hospital in Los Angeles, the doctor suspected that it was cancer. So I immediately went to cancer specialized hospital for CT examination. The final diagnosis was large intestine cancer. At that time, the cancer had grown to the late state and I had to receive an operation immediately. Since my wife is Chinese, my mother-in-law sent to me Tian Xian liquid, a kind of traditional Chinese medicine welcome in Hong Kong as I was waiting for the operation. The operation was very successful. Although the tumor was removed, a few cancer cells still remained in Lymph nodes, which would likely lead to another attack. So I received chemical treatment and at the same time, drank Tian Xian liquid. The doctor said that radiation and chemical treatment are likely to cause side-effects like vomiting, weakening of strength, hair-dropping, etc. Fortunately, no side-effect occurred to me.

Afterwards, I continued to drink Tian Xian liquid. As a result, the cancer cells left after the operation were completed eliminated and did not attack again. But during the half a year after the operation, my weight dropped over 50 kg. But now it has returned to the original 78 kg and I work even more energetically than before.

My family consists of 8 people (my wife, four children and parents) and I have to work for another five or ten years. To prevent another attack and enhance health, I drink two bottles of Tian Xian liquid for me and my family.

Changing crisis to chances of life

Lin Sufeng Taiwan middle school teacher 54

In February, 1998, I suddenly had terrible diarrhea and my weight dropped 8 kg for no reason. Finally due to the blooding of anal opening, I went to hospital for examination and the diagnosis was large intestine cancer.

According to the doctor, "having blood in the stool is the characteristic symptom of large intestine cancer. So even if the blood comes from haemorrhoids, you should go to hospital for check. Many take it for granted that the blood in stool is haemorrhoids so that the detection of large intestine cancer is delayed." When I was diagnosed as having large intestine cancer, I underwent an operation immediately. Before the operation, my colleague introduced Tian Xian liquid to me. in fact, I heard that the wife of my colleague had her breast cancer cured for drinking Tian Xian liquid. So I began to drink it without hesitation.

After reading materials about Tian Xian liquid, I came to know that quite a few people are drinking Tian Xian liquid all over the world, which enhanced my confidence in it. I thought that only Tian Xian liquid could save me. After the operation began the radiation and chemical treatment. At the same time I took Tian Xian liquid and Tian Xian pills, which obviously mitigated the side-effect of radiation and chemical treatment.

Compared with other patients who were hospitalized for the same disease and symptoms, I recovered much more quickly. Six months later, the examination showed that everything was in normal condition. I will continue to take Tian Xian liquid and Tian Xian pills from now on.

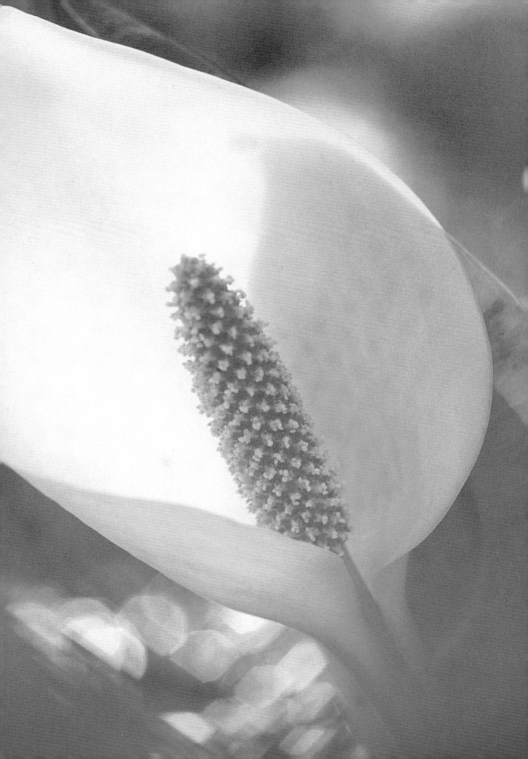

Experiences of defeating prostate cancer successfully

A surprising delight in returning to life miraculously

Mr Sakui   Kanagawa County director of a company   77

I underwent an operation on rectum cancer in 1992 and recovered well. I lived an energetic life in the following seven years.

However, the year before last, I began to have haenaturia and was suspected to suffer from prostate cancer. The doctor told me helplessly, "Even an operation on prostate will not help." In February that year, I was sent to hospital by an ambulance for intestinal obstruction. I had thought myself very healthy and never expected another attack. From then on, I began to fight against cancer. Two months later, in the middle of April, I was faced with a choice whether to undergo another operation or wait for death. Finally I decided to face death in natural way. An operation was not possible, since the cancer cells had transferred to the marrow. But I did not want any harm done to my body.

As I decided to face death, cancer cells invaded my whole body at surprising speed. I was weakening day by day. At that time, whatever treatment for cancer I heard of, I would like to have a try, including pipa acupuncture. Then I finally heard of Tian Xian liquid and began to drink it on August, 10. Out of my expectation, the weakening strength recovered gradually day by day! "Does it mean I have returned to life miraculously?" The hope that I dared not think of returned to me and I continued to drink it. Although I had accepted death, I still did not refuse all other treatment. So at the same time, I underwent radiation treatment in possible range.

It did take effect after one or two months. I felt as if I were another person. My strength was recovering. The cancer neither transferred nor grew.

In greeting the millenium, I designed a card and sent it to declare that I was still alive. Those relatives and friends were all surprised. Anyway I am still a patient. In spring, I catch a cold and have a fever or feel weak occasionally. Thus I will drink more Tian Xian liquid. I believe that I am sure to defeat cancer.

Strength is the source of life and I will do more than ordinary people to enhance my strength.

Regain the happiness of life

Mr Kanada Tokyo jobless 81

In January, 1991, I underwent an operation for stomach cancer and had two thirds of the stomach cut off. Although endoscope could also take out the part with cancer cells, I still chose operation to have the tumor removed once for all. I recovered well after the operation and thought that since the cancer was detected early, I did not have to worry about the transfer or another attack.

In July that year, I was found to have prostate cancer and it was suspected to have transferred to bladder and deteriorated terribly. Due to my old age, the doctor did not suggest an operation but radiation treatment and the injection of hormone.

At that time, I did not hope to defeat cancer completely, but I was still worried whether the treatment could solve the problem or it could only control the spreading of cancer cells. I felt very uneasy. Most of the patients around me did not undergo operation but received radiation or chemical treatment. Although the disease was under control temporarily and turned better, but they died one or two years later.

At that time, I found the book "Fighting against Cancer". There are numerous books and advertisements about cancer in market, however, I couldn't tell why I was so attracted by the book. Of course, it is about Tian Xian liquid. I think I am very lucky. After reading the book, I was not doubtful at all and began to drink Tian Xian liquid. At the beginning of September, radiation treatment started. I called the Japanese branch of International Cancer Recovery Association for consultation, and they suggested me not eating Tian Xian pills during this period of time. So I drank six bottles of Tian

Xian liquid per day and in the middle of October, began to use Tian Xian suppository before going to bed.

In radiation treatment, I neither felt pain nor itching. But since it worked on my abdomen, I had serious diarrhea. For several days, I had to go to toilet over ten times per day. Except for diarrhea, I did not feel other side-effect, nor tired.

I was not sure whether it was the effect of Tian Xian liquid, since radiation treatment and the drinking of Tian Xian liquid began at the same time. Besides, I was not free of the side-effect because of Tian Xian liquid.

The radiation treatment continued 33 times and finished at the end of October. The PSA (tumor indicator) dropped from 120 to 100 after ten days' treatment and to 70 at the beginning of November after the treatment was finished. At that time, I had drunk Tian Xian liquid for one and a half months.

Afterwards, I began to take hormone at the beginning of November and PSA dropped sharply to 20 at the end of the month. The tumor reduced in size and could hardly be felt through palpation. The doctor who was rather surprised than delighted told me the result of the examination excitedly. I was convinced that it was the dual effects of western treatment and traditional Chinese medicine. The quick change of symptoms even surprised the doctor.

The uneasiness that had been haunting me for a long time eventually disappeared and I felt relieved for the first time. More important, I felt the happiness of "life".

During this period, I reported my experiences to the Japanese branch of International Cancer Recovery Association and inquired about the subsequent treatment. So at the beginning of December, I began to eat six Tian Xian pills per day.

Afterwards, the disease turned better more quickly. PSA dropped to 1.5 in January 2000, to 0.6 in February, to 0.4 in March and to the lowest level of 0.1 in April. Even the doctor couldn't help feeling excited, "it can't drop even lower. So great! keep such state. Go on."

I am not sure whether the quick recovery was all due to the treatment of western medicine, neither can I say that it was owning to Tian Xian liquid, since I underwent the treatment of western medicine and drank Tian Xian liquid at the same time. However, one thing is sure. That is, the quick recovery is the real fact. I think without the help or Tian Xian liquid, I would not have recovered so quickly.

I am finally convinced that cancer is by no means terrible as long as we stick to drinking Tian Xian liquid. It has been one year since I was found to have cancer. The cancer cells in bladder also disappeared. The possible transfer to pelvis did not occur.

I believe it is due to Tian Xian liquid that I can live every comfortable day now. In the future, I will regulate the amount and continue to drink it.

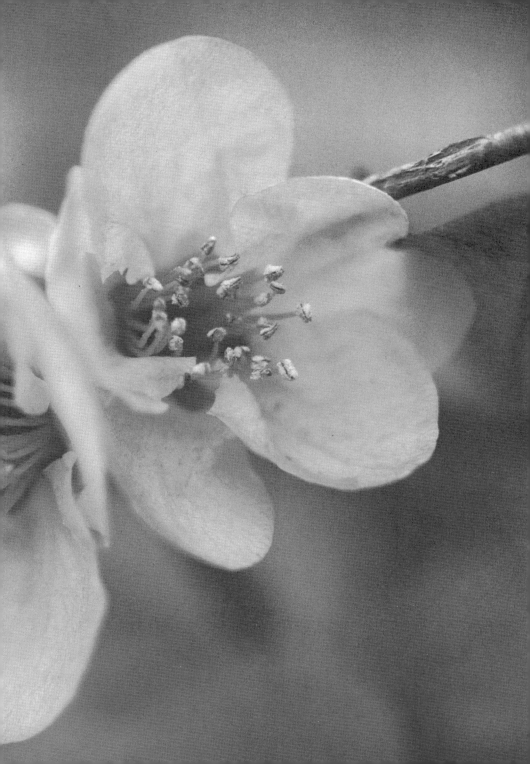

Experiences of defeating malignant lymph tumor successfully

Experiences in fighting against cancer four times

Lady Matsuda housewife 57

In 1993, I was sent to hospital for ovary cancer and underwent an operation and anti-cancer treatment. Although my strength recovered and life returned to normal soon, in June, 1995, I felt great pain in the back and coughed terribly, unable to eat food. The examination in the nearby public hospital showed that I suffered from malignant lymph tumor in the lymph nodes around the stomach. Then I received treatment of anti-cancer drug for six months and it was during this period that I came to know Tian Xian liquid through news report.

The report told that a cancer patient at the late stage in Chuan Yue Dai Jing San hospital turned better after drinking Tian Xian liquid. After reading it, I immediately decided to have a try. I obtained the detailed information and began to drink it in October. Since I stayed in hospital at that time, I sought doctor's advice, "since it also aims at curing cancer, you can have a try." So I decided to bet on the expected effect and finished the treatment.

In April next year, I was hospitalized three months for receiving the transplant of bone stem cells and the treatment of anti-cancer drug. Of course, I didn't stop drinking Tian Xian liquid.

Although I knew beforehand that the side-effect of anti-cancer drug would lead to loss of appetite, hair-dropping and the doctor also told me directly that "transplant of bone stem cells equals treatment of large-amount anti-cancer drug", I suffered a lot from the violent side-effect for I underwent two kinds of treatment at the same time. At first, I constantly felt sick and unable to take in food. "Have I gone to the end of life?" Death occurred in my mind repeatedly! However, compared with those patients younger than me around 40, my recovery was much quicker and I myself couldn't believe it. Afterwards, the side-effect of anti-cancer drug made me feel lull in hands and feet. After I lived a normal life for one year, tumor was again found in my pelvis in August, 1997 without any obvious symptom. I had to undergo an operation and the treatment of anti-cancer drug in hospital.

The treatment finished and I was released from hospital in January, 1998. The tumor indicator was 110 at that time. The doctor said that when it rose up to 150, I should go to hospital to receive treatment of anti-cancer drug. Since the tumor indicator rose after I left hospital, I asked Mr. Wang for the dosage of Tian Xian liquid and Tian Xian pills and added to the amount according to his instructions. As a result, the tumor indicator dropped gradually to 50 in May. During this period, although tumor indicator was very unsteady, so was my mood, I was still convinced that "it is sure to be cured". I placed all my hope on Tian Xian liquid and Tian Xian pills. Now the tumor indicator has returned to normal.

I have undergone numerous treatments and at the verge of death, only "spirit" could defeat cancer! During my stay in hospital, I was acquainted with many patients but only few have survived. I should not grieve on it. So the most important is "not to hesitate", for we are unable to manipulate our fate and no one could escape death. Therefore, we should enjoy every day in our limited life. In fact, when I made myself happy and delighted, I could feel the surge of strength.

When receiving the treatment of anti-cancer drug, not only did I feel like vomiting, I also suffered from constipation and hair-dropping, but I was still sure that I was able to go through the difficulty.

"Few can still be so energetic like you. So please keep on!" the doctor in charge encouraged me sincerely. This is the basic of treatment.

A friend told me that "disease is not necessarily related to life span". I agree with her. An intimate friend of mine felt nothing wrong at usual time. One day she suddenly fainted for cerebral and thus passed away. But I, a cancer patient, live longer than her. It is a real fact. Now I am very healthy. A few days ago my husband and I had a trip to northern Europe. Life is very long for me!

Symptoms disappear quickly

Kong Chi Keung Hong Kong jobless 77

In the summer two years ago, I suddenly fainted! I was always very strong, so I was quite surprised at the sudden faint. The medical examination in hospital showed dropsy at lung and heart and also found lymph cancer. Due to my old age and weakened strength, the operation had a high risk. Later the doctor told me that the possibility of improvement was less than 20 per cent even with continuous radiation and chemical treatment

During the three months of my stay in hospital, no real treatment was carried out. The symptoms kept deteriorating and weight dropping. In autumn that year, a friend told me of the functions of Tian Xian liquid published in newspaper. After having a deeper understanding of it, my family members bought it.

After I drank it for two months, my weight increased. Chemical treatment began at that time and I still continued to drink Tian Xian liquid. As we know, chemical treatment would lead to hair-dropping and loss of appetite, but neither my hair dropped, nor did I lose appetite, I did not feel like vomiting either.

Since I have been working in fiber factory and later in gas station, the doctor said the cancer might have something to do with working in gas station. But seeing me work so energetically in my seventies, he couldn't say more. Soon afterwards, the examination in December showed that the lymph cancer reduced to unbelievable size and I could obviously feel the improvement of my physical state. So I was eager to leave hospital.

Now I also use Tian Xian suppository. I am surprised as well as happy at my trying new things actively.

Face death courageously

Zeng Yuee Taiwan engaged in processing work 32

Four years ago, a lump of the size of a peanut appeared in my throat. As it grew bigger, my voice turned more and more hoarse. So I went to Chang Gen hospital near my home for check and I was told that it was a benign tumor. An operation was performed immediately to have it removed. Afterwards, although I underwent chemical treatment continuously, my strength did not recover and I felt worse.

I am a divorced professional woman with a six-year-old daughter and a nine-year-old son. Considering the future of my children, I hoped that the doctor could tell me the real fact. Then I knew that I suffered from malignant lymph tumor. It was the fourth month after the operation. My mine was in emptiness. I even thought of dying with my children together!

Like a nightmare I would never wake from

A friend who studies traditional Chinese medicine told me of Tian Xian liquid after he knew of my disease and sent the liquid for me to drink one month.

I began to drink Tian Xian liquid when I underwent chemical treatment. About half a year later, the effect showed up. I believed it was due to Tian Xian liquid, so I only relied on it from then on.

Four years have passed. In the examination this January, the doctor said that "cancer cells have all disappeared. The disease is cured." I once gave up the hope to live on, but now, for my two children, I am sure I will live a better life!

Cancer cells disappear quickly

Jian Guodeng Taipei manufacture and sale of automobile parts 42

Such symptoms as headache, vomiting and shaking of body lasted half a year and I went to Taipei central clinic for examination. The doctor made the diagnosis before cerebral haemorrhage attacked me. I was immediately sent to Tai Da hospital to receive an operation. At that time, the lymph cancer had spread and the doctor told the fact to my wife.

But I still thought it was simple cerebral haemorrhage. Two months after the operation, my wife told me the truth. I am always interested in traditional Chinese medicine and believe that slight diseases can be cured by traditional Chinese medicine, so I told myself never to give up.

At that time, a good friend of mine, after knowing my condition, brought me Tian Xian liquid which is said to be effective against cancer.

For a long time, I hoped to cure cancer by traditional Chinese medicine, so I began to drink Tian Xian liquid without hesitation and stopped the radiation and chemical treatment. In the first month, I drank six bottles per day and in the following three months four bottles per day.

Although cancer cells still existed, there was no sign of deteriorating. Besides, the blood circulation was normal, so I didn't feel like a patient.

Of course, I continue to drink Tian Xian liquid and return to work. I have no trouble driving the bus and I believe cancer will be cured in another one or half a year.

For myself and my wife, never to give up

Huang Qingbiao food processing Taiwan 37

In April, 1997, hard lumps appeared in throat and under left armpit. After the examination in the nearby hospital, it was diagnosed as "chronic inflammation". I did not treat it seriously.

Half a year later, hard lumps appeared in lymph glands all over my body and my weight kept dropping. So I went to hospital in Taipei for further examination.

The doctor's diagnosis was lymph cancer at the fourth stage. When told the fact, I felt as if in complete darkness, without knowing what to do. Fortunately, my wife's support encouraged me to receive the chemical treatment with violent side-effect. However, vomiting and hair-dropping that came with the treatment greatly tortured me! Although I tried my best to stand the pain of treatment, the marrow test showed that cancer cells had transferred to marrow! My despair was beyond words.

At that time, the colleague in the former company I worked in brought Tian Xian liquid. After his introduction, I began to take Tian Xian liquid and Tian Xian pills and at the same time underwent chemical treatment, though I was still in doubt. In the examinations in May and July of 1998, the doctor in charge told me that "You are very lucky for the cancer cells in marrow are sure to have disappeared almost completely." He attributed it to chemical treatment while I was convinced that it was due to Tian Xian liquid.

Now, although cancer cells keep away from me, the doctor still warns me that the lymph cancer is most likely to attack again, so I should continue to take Tian Xian liquid and Tian Xian pills.

I am very happy that I can recover health and live energetically. Besides, my wife's support, I should thank Tian Xian liquid.

Good products bring new chances

Ma Meiyu   Thailand   housewife   46

I went to hospital for examination for I felt uncomfortable in throat. The doctor's diagnosis was slight inflammation and gave me antiphlogistic. Later on, although the discomfort did not disappear, I did not receive further check for I was busy taking care of children and husband.

In September, 1995, I felt itching at my neck as if stung by mosquito and I scratched it and blood came out. Since the bleeding couldn't be stopped, I went to hospital and was found to have lymph tumor! An operation was performed the second month to cut off two of the three tumors. The other one could not be cut off for it was near the artery.

Fortunately, since my husband works in a government department, we live a better off life and could afford to take traditional Chinese medicine when I underwent chemical treatment. We got information about traditional Chinese medicine on internet and knew Tian Xian liquid. So I went to the drugstore in Bangkok and it happened to sell Tian Xian liquid. However, after I drank it, although there was sign of improvement, the pain grew more acute and the symptoms deteriorated. Even now I can still feel my disappointment! I did not have the strength to go to the drugstore to protest.

One day, I happened to see reports about Tian Xian liquid in Hong Kong newspaper. I thought "Maybe I have been cheated?" I compared the package of Tian Xian liquid in the photo of the newspaper with that I bought. They are really different! Besides, what was described in the newspaper was also different from my condition. After my husband inquired Hong Kong news agency, I was sure that the Tian Xian liquid I bought from Tang Ren Street was forged! The Hong Kong newspaper also said that forged Tian Xian liquids are countless. Besides, I confirmed that there are cases that the real Tian Xian liquid cured cancer.

After I got the telephone number of the general agency of China No.1 Tian Xian liquid, I placed an order directly from Hong Kong. The Tian Xian liquid sent from Hong Kong was the same as the one in the newspaper. This is the real Tian Xian liquid. As I expected, the effect distinguished the real from the forged! The feeling of pain that troubled me most disappeared after I drank it for a month. Half a year later, the lymph tumor reduced in size. Since I also underwent chemical treatment, the effect could not be wholly attributed to Tian Xian liquid. But I dared say that Tian Xian liquid was absolutely effective.

As I thought I had recovered enough, I stopped drinking Tian Xian liquid and only relied on chemical treatment. Immediately my strength weakened, the disease deteriorated and the feeling of pain returned to me. The examination showed that the tumor grew in size. I picked up drinking Tian Xian liquid again. After this experience, I know I will not stop drinking Tian Xian liquid until I have really recovered.

Now I rely on Tian Xian liquid and, according to my physical condition, use Tian Xian suppository too. The lymph tumor has reduced and can't be felt by hand.

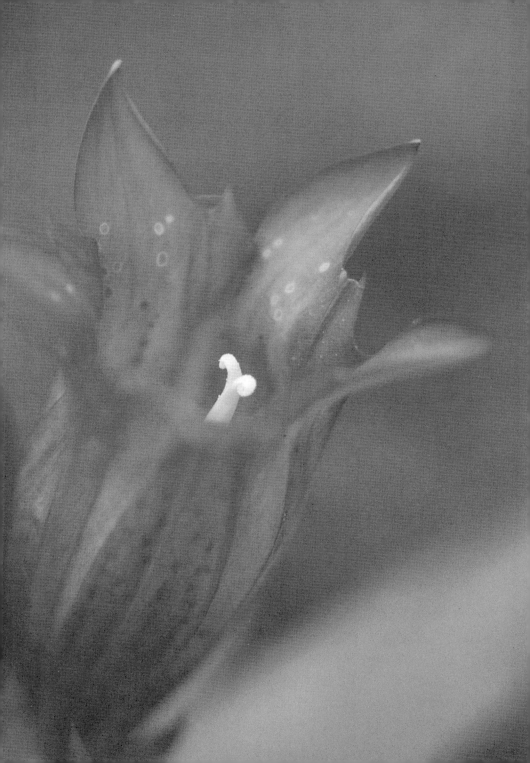

Experiences of defeating skin cancer

Family members' support surpasses all

Lady Nagada Gifu County   housewife   49

In August, 1995, I was found to have skin cancer at neck (malignant melanoma). I have fought against the disease for five years up till now.

In the first two years after the operation, I was on the mend and returned to my normal life except for the regular examination in hospital. Unexpectedly, the examination in the third year showed that the cancer cells transferred to chest. Afterwards, I received the treatment of anti-cancer drug and at the same time I tried all other medicines available including Chinese caterpillar fungus. But nothing brought exciting effect. As I was at a loss, I came to know Tian Xian liquid from the program "Sheng Dao HIROSI Good morning" on radio and advertisement in newspaper and I bought it immediately.

In the first three months, I drank four bottles of it per day. After cancer cells were found to have transferred to abdomen, I ate six Yian Xian pills in addition. Fortunately, the tumor in chest reduced in size. Although the tumor in abdomen remained unchanged, the disease was finally put under control.

When the cancer cells were found to have transferred to the bone of my leg, I began to take six bottles of it per day and twelve Tian Xian pills and underwent radiation treatment.

I couldn't do housework even with the crutch. Without the support of my family, I couldn't have got through! Not only my husband, three children of mine also pay great attention to my condition. They search for anti-cancer medicines and health food from internet and advertisements and do housework for me. My gratitude to my family is beyond words.

Now, I hope to share the experiences and feelings with other patients who suffer from malignant melanoma. Besides communication with family members, more ideas and suggestions would be exchanged if a meeting could be held for people who drink Tian Xian liquid.

Determine to exist with cancer

Mr Amenaka Chiba County   obless 71

Twelve or thirteen years ago, skin cancer was found on my ring finger. Since I always held a conservative attitude towards western medicine, so after seeking consultation with experts, I decided to adopt the treatment of traditional Chinese medicine, dieting, Qi Gong, acupuncture and moxibustion.

The cancer at the initial stage was most difficult to deal with as if mocking at me who underwent treatment seriously. The cancer cells spread to both hands and three months later I felt as if they spread through my whole body. The left wrist that cancer attacked first swelled to double the size and I felt piercing pain in every part of my body.

Afterwards, cancer appeared in internal organs like breast cancer and kept deteriorating. Of course I tried my best to fight against it. I told myself that cancer would not take my life away but existed with me.

However, the real fact was much more serious. I was in cold sweat for the tremendous pain in abdomen, but I could do nothing but bear it.

Two years ago, I got to know Tian Xian liquid and began to drink it. After I analyzed its ingredients and studied it thoroughly, I was convinced that I was to be saved.

As I expected, I felt warm in my body and excited.

One year and a half have passed. I, who is quite critical of traditional Chinese medical science and medicine, continue to drink Tian Xian liquid. I am the best testimony.

In the past, I was afraid to have a trip to other places for I suffered from the great pain all over my body. But now I am free of it. The recent examination shows that the functions of my internal organs have improved. All this is due to Tian Xian liquid.

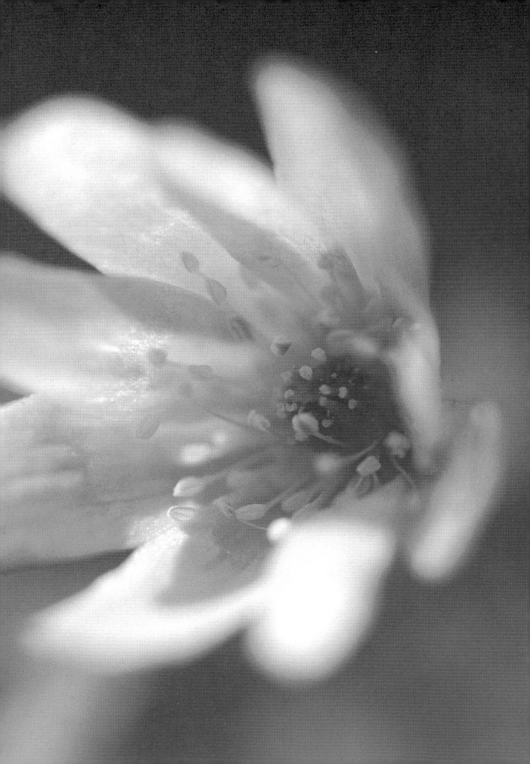

Experiences of defeating bone cancer

Defeat the tremendous pain caused by cancer

Lady Nagada   Shijuoka   County   housewife   69

After the physical examination in 1989, I underwent an operation for I suffered from undifferentiated cancer in right thyroid gland and continued to take hormone up till now. Although life returned to normal afterwards, five years later, in 1994, cancer appeared in uterus and another operation was performed to cut it off. However, one year later, remaining cancer cells were found in vagina and I underwent the third operation.

The last operation to cut off the remaining cancer cells was a big accident! I thought it was the fault in the operation for, at that time the bladder had adhered to the intestine and the operation cut off the healed bladder. As a result, urine flowed to the abdomen and bladder got deteriorated. The doctor suggested cutting off the whole bladder, but I hoped to keep at least the half. Finally a small part was left.

Only this operation could cause a great burden to the body. In September, 1998, the cancer was found to have transferred. At first, I felt slight pain in the back and waist. Subsequently, the acute pain made me unable to move. I was sent to hospital and the doctor said that the operation on the waist might make me unable to walk. Considering that I was approaching 70, I refused the operation and received radiation treatment.

However, the pain in my waist was not relieved although treatment was carried out. I could neither sit nor stand. And I had difficulty in turning over even if I lay down. I took morphine to kill the pain during my stay in hospital and continue it after I was released from hospital. But it did not solve the problem!

At that time, my daughter's friend gave me a book entitled "Fighting against Cancer". "You'd better try other medicines than wait for death." Supported by my family, I began to drink Tian Xian liquid for five months as I was bedridden. Gradually the pain was mitigated and I no longer needed to add to the dosage of morphine. Finally I could walk around without being supported by others. Sometimes I even forgot to take morphine.

It was really unbelievable, wasn't it? In September, 1998, my family members were still afraid that I could spend the new year with them, but now I was able to greet the millenium with my beloved family. Now I am energetic! Although I can't hold one posture for long, I am able to do some housework. Before I fell ill, I was tired of cooking the three meals, washing clothes and cleaning the room every day. But now I feel delighted at one thing I can do well. I can take interest in weaving and patching. Considering the design of the pattern, I am really satisfied.

Going through such a terrible disease, I think one's fate is destined. Of course I hope to live longer. Besides, after drinking Tian Xian liquid, I no longer feel anxious but more vigorous to challenge new things. However, one shouldn't demand too much of himself. Keep optimistic, relax yourself and you will be strong enough to fight against disease.

I am not the only one who suffers from cancer

Lady Yamamura   Kanagawa County   housewife   65

It was seven or eight years ago that I came to know Tian Xian liquid because of my husband's disease.

Several years after we forgot Tian Xian liquid, in the regular examination, the doctor said that "the tumor indicator rises obviously so you need to undergo drip feeding". So I received the injection of drip feeding for three hours. After that, my husband said, "Let's go back home after taking the medicine". Out of expectation, the medicine I held in my hand was anti-cancer drug.

I went to hospital one week later and asked the doctor in a trembling voice, "Have I caught cancer?" This was the first time that I heard of "poly-myeloma". At that time, I thought that if I really caught cancer, I should drink Tian Xian liquid.

In October, Tian Xian liquid I place an order for was sent to me through the agency. After drinking it for some time, the sense of lull in my feet and hands turned better.

In the Spring Festival, my daughter and I planned to take my 3-year-old grandson to visit the Palace Museum in Taiwan. About one week before the trip, I underwent the injection of drip feeding in hospital and took medicine. I brought Tian Xian liquid with me. Although all my hair dropped after I returned from Taiwan, I had a nice trip anyway. I thought that Tian Xian liquid mitigated the side-effect, so I encouraged myself constantly.

Soon afterwards, with excitement, I took part in the meeting for exchange in Tokyo organized by the Japanese branch of International Cancer Recovery Association. After listening to the speeches delivered by Mr. Wang and the warm-hearted Mr. A Bu from the ninth clinic as well as the real experiences in fighting against cancer, I found I was not the only one fighting against cancer. There were so many people of strong character and will power trying their best to defeat cancer.

Now, I no longer feel lull in hands and feet and the tumor indicator gets steady. I used to go to hospital once a week, but now once a month. Next year I am going to Kampuchea to visit the Wu Ge Burrow, so I am full of expectation and excitement. In order to control the side-effect, I continue to drink four bottles of Tian Xian liquid besides acupuncture and moxibustion.

I am filled with gratitude to Tian Xian liquid.

Return to life miraculously when there are only 3 months' life left

Mr Klarkon   South Africa college professor   57

I was found to have myeloma with my friend Dr. Botag's examination! I though it could be cured with treatment. However, the follow-up examination in April, 1995 showed that myeloma attacked again. "I am sorry to say that the cancer has transferred to the hand, and you can only live for three to six months."

Although I could accept the fact, but could not stand the tears of my family members and the desperate expressions in their eyes. As I gave up and began to arrange my work and spend more time with my family, in July, my elder brother, who was dispatched to work in the embassy in India sent me a letter with report about Tian Xian liquid and emphasized that I should have a try. I did not cherish any hope, but only wanted to leave more time to my family, so I decided to drink it.

Since it took to order and mail, it was already in August that I began to drink it. Wonder was achieved! One or two weeks later, my weakened strength gradually recovered.

In another examination, even Dr. Botag was surprised at my recovery. And all kinds of tests showed improvement. The examination in May, 1997 found that cancer cells disappeared. The regular marrow test and blood test also show that everything is quite normal.

It is the real miracle achieved with me! The doctor once predicted that I could live six months but I have survived. I believe that since I can recover, others can, too. Never give up life and believe in the effect and hope brought by Tian Xian liquid.

My experience about bone cancer

Wan Rsbiatul Malacca student 13

In October, 1998, I found my left leg a little swollen. At that time, I was going to take part in the sports meet in Wu Ji Zhi Na Area on school level on behalf of my school and often practiced playing the ball and 100-meter hurdle race. So I thought that I had my leg sprained. However, as the sports meet was approaching, my left leg was swollen more and more. It seemed that I couldn't take part in the sports meet on behalf of my school. I told what happened to my parents. My father did not take it seriously and mother also attributed it to sprain.

Two or three days later, my mother sent for a massage doctor to help me, but it did not work at all. Later, mother took me to some private clinic and the doctor only gave me some anti-biotic medicine for detumescence. Since it still did not work, mother took me to the same clinic and the doctor told her to take me to Malacca central hospital to take an X-ray photo. It turned out that the cancer had deteriorated and I was told to be hospitalized immediately. However, Malacca does not have the equipment to diagnose and treat cancer, I was transferred to Kuala Lumpur Ma Da Medical Center.

There the doctor carried out CT scan and test on me to confirm the disease. After all examinations were done, the diagnosis was bone cancer. According to the result of the examinations, the doctor decided to carry out chemical treatment first, followed by an operation. The chemical treatment lasted six courses, three before the operation and another three after it.

All my hair dropped, including eyebrows and eyelashes. To avoid the sunshine, which made my eyes uncomfortable, I had to wear sunglasses. All the sufferings, I believed, were the way that led me to recovery with the help of God, as people say.

On December, 31, 1998, I was sent to the operation room with the company of my parents, brother and sister to undergo the operation on left leg. I was very afraid at that time, felt an impulse to run away, but I couldn't. Then, I lost consciousness. When I opened my eye again, I saw my parents and siblings sit by the bedside, so I did not sense anything wrong to me. It was until three days later that I found my left leg cut off. I cried and shouted like a mad. How could I face others for I had been maimed. On the fourth day after the operation, I understood that I could do nothing but accept the fact, face the reality courageously and learn to walk with the help of crutch.

On March, 15, 1999, I was diagnosed as lung infection and in the CT scan, the doctor found two small tumor in my left lung and one in the right one. I was greatly surprised and frightened. However, I had learned to suppress my feelings. The doctor suggested an operation to my parents and it had a high risk. But without the operation, the chance of survival was very slight, for the cancer cells in my body were very active and spread quickly. Besides, the operations should be performed in a short period of time. In other words, the operations on the left and right chests should be done within a week. My parents let me make the decision myself. Considering my health, I agreed to the doctor's suggestion of operation.

One week later, and I still remember clearly it was April, 14, 1999, I was sent into the operation room again. However, due to my weakened physique and constant coughing, the doctor thought it not the time for an operation. It was not until April 21 to 28 that the operations on my chest were successfully performed. Seven small tumors were cut off from my left lung and nine from my right lung. These tumors were too small to be measured. Chemical treatment continued and I returned to hospital for blood test after the course was finished.

In December, 1999, the doctor suspected that the cancer cells might have spread to heart and prepared me to undergo supersonic check. I was put in the double ward. My roommate was a girl who suffered from blood cancer. One that day, the girl's uncle, who is a Chinese visited her. He said to my mother, "As to your daughter's disease, I once took part in a relevant speech that introduced an effective traditional Chinese medicine. Next time I will bring the address of the agency to you." Several hours later, I was called to have the heart examination, but the doctor couldn't find any cancer cell in my heart, as he expected. The next day, that Chinese uncle brought the address of the agency of the medicine. However, he seemed a little hesitant about its price. That afternoon, mother asked for the permission for me to leave hospital, then she went to see the agency of the medicine directly and asked about the detailed information. At home my disease got worse, so I had to be sent to hospital again. The effort to save money to buy the Chinese medicine was stopped.

Finally, in December, mother bought China No.1 Tian Xian liquid and No.5 Tian Xian pills. After I took the medicine four months, I went to hospital for another examination. The doctor said that the tumors in my lung were not active, nor did they grow. However, it should be proved by X-rays. In June, 2000, I was again called to have another X-ray check (the second time in the same day), for the doctor said he could not believe the result of the first one. So he showed the second photographic plate to a professor. The professor thought that it couldn't be said that the tumors in my body were completely eliminated, but the doctor argued that my lung appeared clear the X-ray photo. So when the X-ray analyst got the photographic plate, he couldn't believe the report either and had to resort to Prof. Peads Klinik, who agreed with the doctor. In order to confirm it, in July, I had another X-ray check. The result proved what the doctor said as unbelievable and the professor described as very special. The good news brought some laughter to my family and I also hoped that it was true.

Up till now, I have taken Tian Xian liquid and Tian Xian pills for five months. I can go to school with the help of crutch, my weight rises to 43kg and I have done a good job of study. Although I did not go to school for a year, I still passed UPSR examination. Here I'd like to express sincere gratitude to China No.1 Tian Xian liquid and No.5 Tian Xian pills which gave me the confidence and happiness to live on.

May China No.1 Tian Xian liquid and No.5 Tian Xian pills bring me a bright future for ever!

October 2000

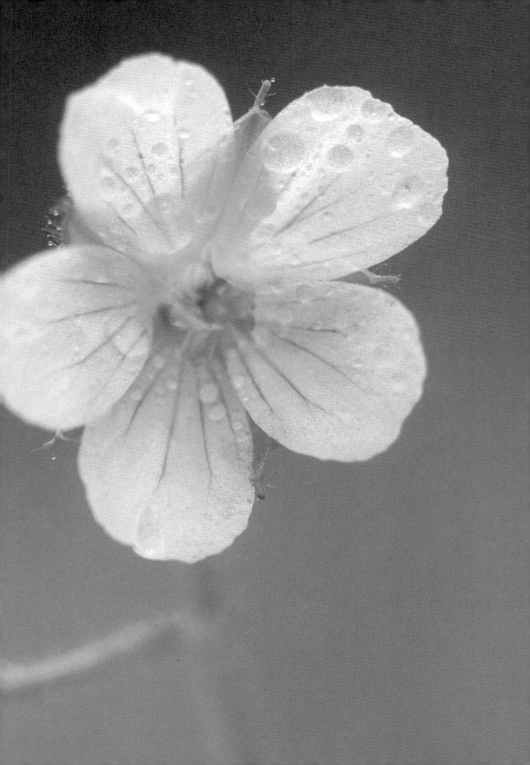

Experiences of defeating laryngopharyns cancer successfully

Try in various ways and strengthen confidence

Mr Nakahara Igeraki County jobless 64

It is over one year since I began to drink Tian Xian liquid. In March, 1999, the doctor declared that I had laryngopharyns cancer, so my wife searched for books about cancer, among which I was attracted by one book entitled "Fighting against Cancer". I began to take eight bottles of Tian Xian liquid and nine Tian Xian pills before I finished reading the book.

The laryngopharyns cancer is at the entrance of the esophagus about 1 cm wide and 2.5 cm long. It was planned that I was to undergo an operation after the tumor was reduced in size by the radiation treatment.

However, during the period of radiation treatment, I discussed with my family the life after operation and view of value and finally we decided not to receive the operation, but only rely on radiation treatment to prevent the tumor from deteriorating, and after that, place all hope on Tian Xian liquid and Tian Xian pills. For compared with other patients, the side-effect of radiation treatment on me was obviously more slight

In other words, there was no scald of the skin or loss of appetite. I could take in food and did not need to receive the injection of drip feeding. I only had slight scald and little change of vocal cords, which recovered naturally after the treatment. Both the doctors and nurses were surprised. In fact., I received more amount of radiation (76 Gray) than all the other patients and it continued 42 days. However, during the nearly 80 days' stay in hospital, I ate meals every day without exception.

It is said that when the amount of radiation surpasses 30, many people could not walk but rely on drip feeding for survival. It is due to Tian Xian liquid that I could be relieved of the side-effect.

Precious as Tian Xian liquid is, I still felt a little unwell as I began to drink it, so I had to add to or reduce the dosage when necessary. Now I take four bottles of Tian Xian liquid per day and twelve Tian Xian pills. As the treatment began, the doctor said that "only operation can cure the disease". Of course I do not forget the doctor's words, but I decide to bet on Tian Xian liquid. Now neither CT, MRI examinations show anything wrong, nor is there any sign of transfer. Although I bear what the doctor said in mind, yet more do I believe in the choice my wife made after her careful consideration. I will continue to drink Tian Xian liquid with confidence in the future.

Resolution of never giving up

Mr Tanaka Saga County owner of a private enterprise 64

In February, 1996, the local hospital diagnosed me as suffering from laryngopharyns cancer and I was sent to hospital immediately. I underwent the treatment of anti-cancer drug to reduce the size of the tumor and then an operation was performed.

I felt well after the operation and was released from hospital in April. Before I could enjoy the happiness of recovery, I felt great pain at the end of September. The examination in hospital showed that cancer cells attacked again and the doctor said that I could only rely on radiation treatment this time.

Soon afterwards, the neighbour who was drinking Tian Xian liquid recommended it to me. So I began to drink it and at the same time underwent chemical treatment.

I drank six bottles of Tian Xian liquid per day. Three months later, the pain stopped and the tumor disappeared! The doctor also said that "there is no sign of transfer". Now, I am in good mental and physical state and invulnerable to cold. More important, I can enjoy a healthy life. I still continue to drink Tian Xian liquid to make me feel at ease.

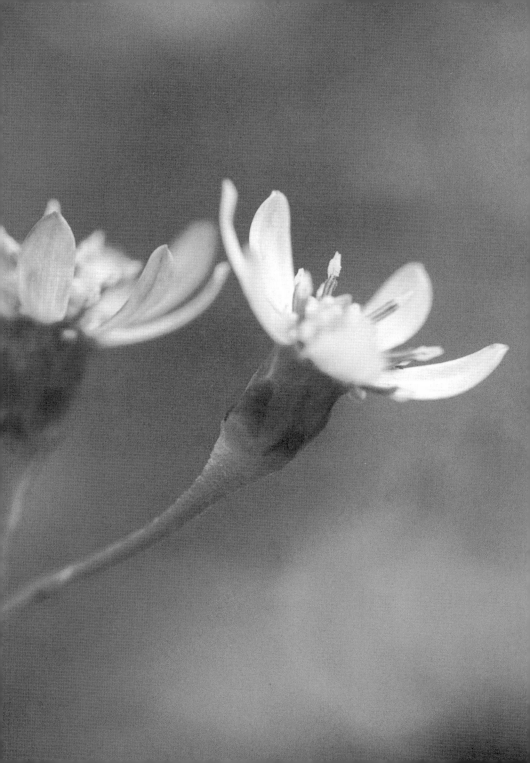

Experiences of defeating thyroid gland successfully

Feel the essence of never giving up

Mr Ikeyama Yamanashi County employee of a company 41

It is ten years since thyroid gland was found

At first I underwent the operation to have the thyroid gland cut off. Eight and a half years passed and cancer cells were again found in lung, brain and neck. I underwent another operation immediately. Soon the cancer cells were found to have transferred to the two lungs and the doctor told me that I could only live three or four years.

At that time, I was only 30 years old and couldn't give up out of fear. After the operation, I tried all means effective against cancer, including dieting treatment with the help of my wife.

In May, next year, cancer was found in the lymph gland at my neck and I underwent an operation to have it cut off and in July another operation was performed to cut open the wind tube that made breathing difficult.

I am fond of delicious food, so dieting treatment caused some pain to me. Besides, due to the pressure that work exerted on me, sometimes I couldn't pay attention to too much. I was quite depressed. In August, I suffered from pneumonia and had blood in phlegm out of no reason and was sent to hospital for hypercalcinemia. My weight dropped from 65 kg before the second operation to 45 kg and I was weakened a lot.

Once strength was lost, various symptoms occurred one after another

As soon as pneumonia was cured, my voiced turned hoarse in winter. In February, next year, as I was going to undergo isotope radiation treatment to prevent another attack, blood phlegm occurred again. Frankly speaking, I thought I was going to die! No effect was achieved whatever I tried! Were there no other ways besides radiation treatment? At that time, I thought of Tian Xian liquid.

I bought books and placed an order to the general agency in Hong Kong. At that doubt I was quite doubtful of the reports about the recovered patients and 80 percent effect, and thought that they were only for promotion.

There are numerous cases that consumers are cheated by various kinds of health food in market, including traditional Chinese medicine. However, since isotope radiation treatment did not take much effect, I had to place my hope on Tian Xian liquid. I thought that everyone was going to die, so I plunged myself in work and thus my mood also turned light. Ten days after I began to drink Tian Xian liquid, blood phlegm disappeared and another week later, the pain in my chest also stopped. Besides, my hoarse voice turned better and my complexion became ruddy. Eventually I was able to return to normal work and life. Now my weight is expected to rise to 51 kg and I can go camping for two days and three nights in summer. All this is owed to Tian Xian liquid.

If only I had known Tian Xian liquid earlier

Zhu Zhi Chi   Taiwan orderly 62

I went to many hospitals for diagnosis and treatment. How many people's life is troubled by cancer! I had to go to various hospitals and face various so many doctors. I believed that I could get to know good doctors and good treatments so as to get rid of the monster of cancer.

From the very beginning, doctors' diagnoses were quite unclear. At the beginning of 1995, I went to hospital for examination since I suffered from constant slight coughing but I did not feel anything wrong with the function of my heart. The doctor's diagnosis was asthma and lowering function of heart. However, the treatment did not take effect. One year later, I spit out blood phlegm and went to hospital again, but the cause could not be found. So I had to seek advice from the doctor in the ear-nose-throat section that I was familiar with. The doctor thought my symptom quite strange and introduced me to the chest section in another big hospital and the doctor there diagnosed it as thyroid gland cancer.

That was on January, 16, 1996. I can't remember the details, but only know that I felt complete darkness before my eyes---"I have caught cancer and nothing can help me". I asked my daughter and knew that the doctor said I could only live for three months. My daughter told me firmly that "It is absolutely impossible. We can't wait to die."

First an operation was performed to cut off the thyroid gland and the doctor suspected that the transferred tumor still remained in my body and I had to undergo radiation treatment. So I received treatment in hospital in daytime and went home to sleep. During this time, I did not stop coughing and spitting out phlegm and I gradually lost appetite. Thus every painful day dragged by. At last I couldn't utter sound, so I lost confidence in that hospital.

I consulted the doctor in the ear-nose-throat section, he suggestion having another examination. So I went to the hospital where his teacher worked for check. Although decision had been made at that time to have the throat taken out and a metal duct installed, my daughters and I heard that the operations performed in that hospital all failed! So just before the operation, I left the hospital temporarily on the grounds that my daughter was going to marry and transferred to Buddhism hospital. However, the operation in Buddhism hospital also turned out to be a failure.

When I was sent to hospital at the beginning of September, the doctor said that "after the wind pipe was cut open and the duct was inserted, the voice could be resumed and coughing and phlegm could be stopped." So I underwent the operation. Having lost my voice, I was greatly depressed, for the duct in my throat often came off. And since the lid was not installed at first, the duct even dropped into the bowl when I ate meal. But my family never complained, so I am very grateful to them. My wife and daughters must have shed a lot of tears behind me! At that time, my daughter saw the advertisement of Tian Xian liquid and visited Mr. Xu, the consultant. Now I know that it is Mr. Xu who has saved my life! If it were not for his advice, I could not have resumed my voice.

Mr. Xu is a careful person. He instructed me on how to drink Tian Xian liquid and introduced doctor Gao from the hospital attached Taipei Medical Institute.

Since the hospital attached Taipei Medical Institute carries treatment of western medicine, I did not place much hope. However, doctor Gao is really different from other doctors and the people in the hospital are also kind.

I had to receive radiation treatment for twenty times and I could make sound after the third time and was able to speak after the fifteenth. My vast joy was beyond description. I sincerely felt that life was so nice. It was so unbelievable that I lost my voice for radiation treatment and resumed it also through radiation treatment. It was all due to Tian Xian liquid.

Although cancer cells did not disappear completely, they did not transfer, not spread. And the tumor was found to be reducing in size! My weight rose to 70 kg from the 60 kg after operation.

Not until recently did I know that the doctor once predicted that I could live only three months! My daughter said, " My father, who knows nothing, is so poor." I believe that my wife and children who hide the truth from me suffer much more than me! I tell all my experiences to those who are fighting against cancer but haven't taken Tian Xian liquid. For my family, I will continue to fight.

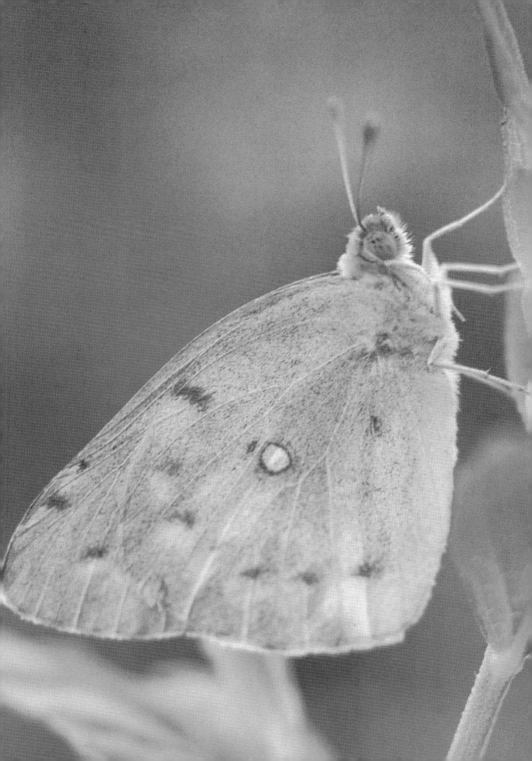

Experiences of defeating nose cancer successfully

I am surprised at the effects of traditional Chinese medicine

Putlachatta Thailand owner of a private enterprise 62

At the beginning of this year, I found a hard lump in my nose. I regarded it as some inflammation and did not pay much attention. Soon, I had increasing difficulty in breathing and went to hospital. The doctor's diagnosis was nose cancer.

The doctor suggested me undergoing radiation treatment for 35 times. My friend recommended Tian Xian liquid to me after knowing its effect. So I began to drink it one week before the treatment and my physical state improved after seven days. I felt the tumor softer than before and breathing unblocked.

I continued to drink Tian Xian liquid when I underwent the radiation treatment. I also took Tian Xian pills to mitigate the side-effect. So I did not feel thirsty and could still work during the time of treatment.

What struck me most was that the tumor really reduced in size after the tenth radiation treatment. After the 28th, the doctor examined and said that "cancer cells disappeared completely. So there is no need for more treatment."

Of course, the doctor was surprised at the drastic change of my disease. I am convinced that my recovery is not due to radiation treatment but Tian Xian liquid.

Find chances of life in despair

Zhou Yuzhen Taiwan carpenter 58

Since the lymph gland behind my ear swelled, I felt it very strange and went to local hospital for examination. The diagnosis was nose cancer.

The doctor said it could be cured in two months after concentrated radiation treatment four or five times. So I accepted the doctor's plan. However, the subsequent treatment not only made me feel pain in nose but dry in throat so that I couldn't fall asleep at night. My weight quickly dropped 10 kg from the original 65 kg. Chemical treatment followed. Five milliliters anti-cancer drug was injected into my body continuously. I felt myself keep weakening. When chemical treatment of fourth months finished, I did not turn better but greatly weakened and I was filled with uneasiness.

At that time, I heard that a friend of mine had his stomach cancer cured after drinking Tian Xian liquid he bought from Hong Kong. So I immediately went to Hong Kong to buy Tian Xian liquid. After I underwent chemical treatment and at the same time drank Tian Xian liquid for two months, my physical state improved. I was very surprised and in the following six months, I only relied on Tian Xian liquid.

It is one year since I was found to have cancer. The examination shows that cancer cells have completely disappeared! The doctor also confirms the effect of Tian Xian liquid and expects me to continue drinking it.

Reproduction of spirit and body

Lee Yuk Yin Hong Kong businessman 52

In April, 1997, my kept weakening for symptoms like cold. I thought it was cold. But I did not recover after two or three months. Soon I found my lymph gland swollen. I was frightened a lot and immediately went to hospital. After the examination was done, the doctor said that it was nose cancer and had transferred to lung and liver. Maybe it was necessary to tell me that I was a cancer patient at the late stage. Since cancer had transferred to lung and liver, I thought I couldn't live long.

Astonished as I was, I was not flurried but received chemical and radiation treatment in hospital under the doctor's instructions. I received radiation treatment six times, and chemical treatment seven times, once per month. But the effect was not satisfactory. The doctor told my wife that I could live for only three months for the cancer was at the late stage. I was not told the truth until later. During this period of time, my wife suffered a lot since the disease improved and deteriorated alternately.

After my knew my disease, a friend once ask me, "do you know Tian Xian liquid?" Since I had no idea of it, I sought the doctor's advice. He said, "how can that sort of thing treat cancer? If you do not trust the hospital, you can leave." We changed a doctor, not that we doubt the former one's ability, but that he was not in the least kind.

From then on, I did not raise any opinions. After radiation treatment and chemical treatment for several times, I did not feel any side-effect that should have shown up. Even the doctor felt it so unbelievable. "Have you taken any other medicine?" "Yes" I did not want to deny, but also did not want explain in detail. The doctor left for he sensed that I did not want to much about it. Three years have passed since the doctor prediction that I could only live for three months. Now I still work on my post.

The regular examination per month shows that the number of white blood cells increases and the size of the lymph tumor reduces. I believe that I have chosen the right treatment. Although the doctor told me that "although the tumor has reduced, it's safer to receive chemical treatment." I do not want to suffer that much.

Now both my physical and mental state has improved. I know my condition best. Although cancer remains unchanged, I believe it will neither grow not deteriorate, but only turn better. My wife finally told me about the doctor's prediction of three months' life, which set both of us laughing. I still live every day well and can do some simple work. I have returned to normal life and feel myself even stronger in spirit. I believe all this is brought by Tian Xian liquid.

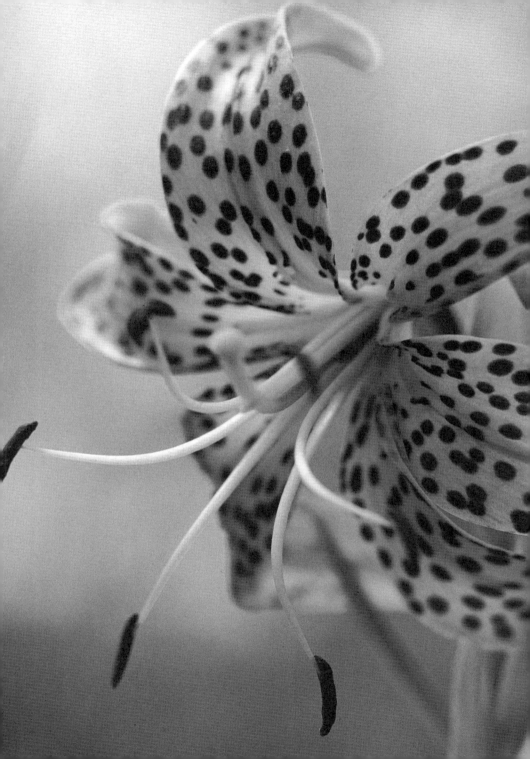

Experiences of defeating esophagus cancer successfully

Regain the happiness from sons and grandsons

Ding Suk Ying   Hong Kong housewife 70

Fifteen years ago I resigned my job and lived a leisure life the company of my grandson. In the autumn three years ago, I felt uncomfortable in throat when I swallowed food and even felt like vomiting after meal. I was suddenly obsessed with a sense of omen.

Nevertheless, I did not take it seriously and gradually I was unable to swallow food. Urged by my daughter, I went to hospital for examination and X-rays showed a tumor in the middle of the esophagus and it was over 10 cm. The doctor said that due to my age, an operation seemed difficult. So he suggested me receiving radiation and chemical treatment.

After the treatment, I was still unable to swallow food. And due to the side-effect, Ii was extremely exhausted to such an extent that I felt like vomiting even when my stomach was completely empty. Maybe I was going to die.

At that time, I came to know Yian Xian liquid, a traditional Chinese anti-cancer medicine from my son-in-law. So I bought it and drank it. To my surprise, two weeks later, I could eat liquid food and in less than a month, the side-effect disappeared and I could eat soft food without difficulty.

The X-ray examination three months later showed that the tumor reduced one third. The doctor said in surprise, "radiation treatment or anti-cancer drug must be quite effective, otherwise how can you recover so quickly?" But I am sure it is due to drinking Tian Xian liquid when I underwent the treatment. Three years have passed and of course, I have fully recovered.

How to take care of the body after operation

Mr Etou Nakashima County employee of a company 40

On August, 6, 1997, I was sent to the hospital attached to the medical department of Jiu Zhou university. In the preceding two months, I had a check in local hospital for there was blood in my urine, but I was released after less than three weeks because the cause was not found. In order detect the disease, I lived in the same hospital again and receive various examinations every day. During this period, I did not take any medicine. On August, 20, a duct was inserted in the ureter and the result was known on August, 28. The doctor in charge told my family members that three tumors were found in the middle part of the left ureter and an operation must be performed to cut off the left kidney and the whole ureter. After more examinations and discussion, the final diagnosis was cancer.

Despite the diagnosis of cancer, my family tried their best to search for various treatments. We got to know information about the treatment for cancer on internet and called Hong Kong directly to place an order. As soon as Tian Xian liquid and Tian Xian suppository arrived, my family members brought it to hospital. On September, 8, I began to use one pill of Tian Xian suppository and drank four bottles of Tian Xian liquid per day. Almost one week later, when the duct was again inserted into the ureter, it was found that the three tumors all disappeared.

The doctor in charge from the hospital attached to Jiu Zhou university had planned a operation cut off the tumors from the bladder and to the bottom of the ureter on September, 16. Due to the effect of Tian Xian liquid, the operation was postponed two weeks and was successfully performed then. I was released from hospital on October, 22.

Now I live every day happily and continue to drink Tian Xian liquid at a lower dosage.

Experiences of defeating tongue cancer successfully

Value Life and Value Tian Xian Liquid

Value life and value Tian Xian liquid Cai Junhui Taiwan bus driver 42

Since I have been driving the long distance from Jiayi and Taipei for a long time, I have to rely on cigarettes and betel nuts to refresh myself. I smoke at least one packet of cigarettes and two packets of betel nuts per day. I still maintain the habit even when I am not driving. As an old saying puts it, "if you often walk at night, you will meet the ghost one day", it does not mean that I have really met the ghost when driving, but that my bad habit--- cigarettes plus betel nuts led me to the monster of tongue cancer.

In 1997, I did not from what time I felt lull and pain on my tongue. So I chewed more betel nuts to make me feel comfortable. One morning, however, when I was cleaning my teeth, I opened my mouth to see it in mirror, only to find that my tongue was different from before. A large part of it was red and black and festering. My heartbeat quickened. I told it to my wife and opened my mouth to let her see. She was also greatly surprised and suggested me asking leave to the company and going to hospital for examination.

She asked her sister to take care of the two children and accompanied me to big hospital in Taipei. Without much check, the doctor told me what disease it was. The purpose of the examination was only to confirm it.

The next day, the doctor made the rounds of the wards, followed by a group of young doctors. He asked me to open my mouth, pointed my tongue to them and let them raise their opinions. Finally he told me that my tongue had to be cut off and the biggest influence was that I would be able to open for my life. Then he went out with the group of young doctors to other wards, leaving my wife and me face to face, without knowing what to do. My wife looked at me, tears flowing down. And before my eyes emerged the scene of me expressing my meanings with my hands. My wife had quarrelled with me many times about my smoking cigarettes and chewing betel nuts, but she did not say anything now. As to me, although I sought the trouble myself, yet it came too early. I was only 42 years old. Cancer only attacked those above 60. Why did it attack me so early?

Anyway, I had to face the reality. I calmed down and told my wife there must be other treatments besides cutting off the tongue. We could ask some friends for relevant information. Eventually, as I stayed at home, waiting for the operation, my sister-in-law brought me a document about China No.1 Tian Xian liquid. I had seen the product in magazine, but I did not trust it because I was born in Taiwan and China No.1 Tian Xian liquid must come from the mainland China. It was reported that many traditional Chinese medicines contain poisonous heavy metal and could not be trusted. So I just put it aside.

However, on thinking that the doctor said that the operation was going to be performed after the results of all examinations were known, my wife took out the document about China No.1 Tian Xian liquid and read it carefully. She urged me to have a try, otherwise there was only one way out---to have the tongue cut off! I agreed to ask my sister-in-law's friend to buy me Tian Xian liquid and Tian Xian suppository which can be squeezed into the anal opening. I thought I'd better follow the instructions since it was very expensive.

Ten days after I took medicine, the doctor informed to go to hospital to prepare for the operation three days later. When the resident physician examined my tongue again, he found that it was different from before. The tongue was more smooth and only a small part was festering. The doctor said the operation should still be performed, but it was not necessary to cut off the whole tongue but the small part. So it would not affect eating and speaking. He asked if I ate traditional medicine these days. I answered directly that I drank China No.1 Tian Xian liquid. He smiled and said that he heard of it and then patted me on the shoulder.

As I was pushed out of the operation room, the doctor told my wife that the bad part had been cut off and it was not big. Care must be taken from now on and smoking and betel nuts must be forbidden. And it's up to you to decide whether to continue to drink Tian Xian liquid. After leaving hospital, I read the introduction about Tian Xian liquid and drank it strictly under the instructions. I went to hospital for check every three months and later half a year. I continue to drink Tian Xian liquid up till now, but do not use Tian Xian suppository and others.

Of course, I dare not smoke or chew betel nuts! I also tell other drivers of the company not to follow me. Anyway, I am filled with gratitude for I can still live a normal life.

Thanks to Tian Xian liquid, I could keep my tongue. I'd like to advise other cancer patients to choose a traditional Chinese medicine to complement the western medicine to achieve better effect and mitigate the pain in

339

treatment.

In fact, I know cancer is likely to attack again, but the chance will be less only if we continue to drink Tian Xian liquid. I make up my mind to accompany my wife and children as long as I can and I won't le the family break down for my sake. I will value every day of my life, as I value every drop of Tian Xian liquid.

Experiences of defeating malignant thymus tumor successfully

There were no side effects even if chemical treatment was carried out

Sing Kam Yuen   Hong Kong   employee of a company   36

I had never expected me to have cancer at my age!

And for some unknown reason, it was malignant thymus tumor, which is rarely seen in the world. In December, 1996, I went to hospital for slight pain in chest and fever. At first, the cause couldn't be detected. After X-rays and various other examinations, it was confirmed to be malignant thymus tumor. The doctor in charge said to me, "there are few such cases in the whole world. Even if the treatment is successfully, it is impossible to recover,"

That it was impossible to recover means that I was near death! Why the doctor told me so directly, I thought, was that he knew I was a Catholic and my belief gave me the courage to face death. But I was frightened and dazed. When I was introspecting the punishment God put on me, I was in great fear of death. When I told my family of my disease, my brother-in-law immediately recommended Tian Xian liquid to me. I thought if western medicine did not help, I could try traditional Chinese medicine. So I began to drink it. During the four months of my stay in hospital, I underwent chemical treatment once a month. However, such side-effects as hair-dropping and vomiting did not happen to me, as I had expected.

Even the doctor was surprised. "It's too marvelous. What's the matter?" I believed that Tian Xian liquid took effect! Another surprise to me was that my girl friend left me when I was released from hospital.

I did not hide the truth from her that I was one without future! However, the idea of marriage to her gave me the strength to fight against cancer. The news that she left me surprised me as much as cancer! But I could not be demoralized. With the notion that God is with me, I continued to receive chemical treatment and at the same time drank Tian Xian liquid.

In May, 1997, the examination at the public hospital showed that cancer cells disappeared. Now, I still go to hospital once a month. That year seemed so long to me. I have used up all the money I saved for marriage. For me with low income, Tian Xoan liquid is really an economic burden.

However, hope exists as long as I survive. I thank Tian Xian liquid for saving my life.

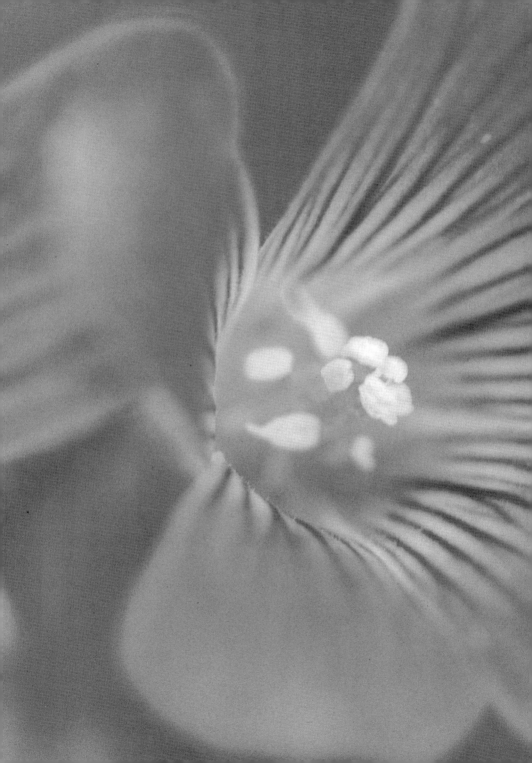

Experiences of defeating other diseases successfully

Family members are surprised at my recovery

Lady Shimitsu   Saitama   County   63

For the whole day, I suffered from diarrhea, acute pain in the back and abdomen, and I felt extremely tired. The doctor diagnosed it as pancreas tumor. It was in the February, this year. The disease was caused by liquid flowing into the pancreas and formed a malign tumor. All the pain was caused by the aftereffect of brain tumor. When the doctor told me the disease, I was too surprised to say anything.

On April, 26, when I was told the result of endoscopy and MRI examination, the doctor also explained the complicated and big operation. I think I will never recall it in my life. Fear and pain tortured me. At that time, I heard of a good traditional Chinese medicine. Although it was not clear whether the medicine could cure the disease, at least I could have a try. My son brought to me the books written by doctor Wang Zhengguo and the information from International Cancer Recovery Association. I originally did not discriminate against traditional Chinese medicine, so I began to acquire a deeper understanding of it.

"Do I have to undergo an operation?" the idea flashed into my mind. So I began to drink Tian Xian liquid from May, 6. The next day, I felt a little different from before. I should continue to drink it. Such was my intuition.

Several days after I drank Tian Xian liquid, the pain in abdomen almost disappeared! One week later, bowel returned to normal. The constant pain also disappeared. Before that, I couldn't sleep well for the pain and when I went out, I always felt upset. My family tried their best to support me.

On May, 29, it was the first time that I went to hospital for the regular MRI examination with excitement.

Two days later, the result came out "the pancreas has obviously reduced in size, so operation is not necessary, but you have to undergo examinations more frequently.

When I heard the result from the doctor and the explanation of the expected operation, I saw the surprised expression on the doctor's face. I knew my condition better than anyone else and I felt more relieved after the doctor confirmed it.

The blood test of outer brain also showed the same result. The doctor said that there was nothing to worry about and even told me to "believe Tian Xian liquid".

In the past I always tried to avoid medical examination in hospital, but now I hope to know the effect of Tian Xian liquid. And on my birthday in October, I also gave a pledge before God to have MRI examination. Recently my son often said, "mother has fully recovered." But I dared relax my vigilance. "It can't be so quick. Be patient."

Besides, the "Shang Rong Tea" that I drank under the instructions of the Japanese branch of International Cancer Recovery Association took much effect against diarrhea. Later on, I came to know that it was also effective for non-cancer patients. So I recommend it to my relatives and friends.

I have drunk Tian Xian liquid for several months. Although I can't give a detailed account here, I will try to tell my experiences to more people and continue drinking it.

Improve physique gradually

Miss Tobashi   Tokyo   employee of a company   26

Two years ago, I went to the gynaecology and obstetrics section of the hospital for the first, for I suffered from dysmenorrhoea constantly when learning in college and now it troubled me a lot in working.

At first, the doctor suspected that it was endometriosis. After various examinations, all doubt was dispelled. The final diagnosis was "period trouble". It began from the pain in back and waist before the period and developed into great headache. During the period, the pain spread through the lower part of my body from abdomen. Besides, I also felt dazed and vomited to the extent that I was unable to walk, but went to and off work by taxi.

The pain-killer given by the hospital had effect for only two or three hours, so did suppository. Since I took the medicine after I felt pain, it caused vomiting and stomachache. So to suppress the stomachache, I had to take other medicine. In this way, my digestive organ had ulcer and bled, and I was hospitalized.

Although I was forbidden to eat and only relied on drip feeding, it was a chance for rest. I suffered a lot from the trouble of digestive organ, and decided not to use pain-killer any longer. Instead, I took up sports like swimming. However, dysmenorrhoea was not a little relieved and I had to endure the monthly pain. At that time, I came across Tian Xian liquid and Tian Xian suppository from the materials I collected.

The traditional Chinese medicines I used to take include agelica and herbaceous peony powder, cassia twig and poris cocos pill, channel warming soup, agelica, etc. I stopped taking some of them for they caused serious diarrhea and others did not take effect after I took them for almost one year. The mystery of traditional Chinese medicine is too profound to understand. "It is not medicine to eat, but if it takes effect, you are very lucky." So I began to use Tian Xian plaster.

I apply Tian Xian plaster to my abdomen, waist, back, etc. On those parts, I neither feel cold or hot, but cool and gradually warm. When the pain aggravates, I apply 8 plasters once and obviously feel the pain mitigated. However, since my skin is very delicate, I feel itching on the part where Tian Xian plaster has been applied and it also turns red. So we should be particularly careful when using Tian Xian plaster in summer.

Although there is no record that Tian Xian suppository is effective against dysmenorrhoea, I still use it according to my own judgement for I have felt its effect. On opening the packet, I smell a special flavour. However, Tian Xian plaster is not small. If you apply one before going to bed, you can have a sound sleep till next morning. During the period, when lying on bed, I bend my waist for the pain. Even if I take pain-killer, the pain will wake me up immediately after the effect of the medicine is gone. So I couldn't sleep at all. Tian Xian plaster is so marvelous!

Although the effect is so satisfactory that the pain disappears after using it. However, I still haven't found the specific drug for dysmenorrhoea. In some months, using Tian Xian plaster and Tian Xian suppository together does not kill the pain. But, the effect is much better than before if I use it according to my physical state.

Anyway, relieving my digestive organ of the burden is the best result to me. It's so nice to find a medicine suitable for me. Some matters of notice should be paid attention to: use Tian Xian suppository three times a day and don't apply Tian Xian plaster to one part over eight hours.

Only those who have suffered from cancer can feel the great pain caused by cancer, so some people do not take dysmenorrhoea seriously, for my pain amounts to nothing compared with that of cancer patients.

However, I have the deepest feeling of pain. It is not only a feeling but exerts a great influence on one's mental state, for one has to endure the pain and does not do want to do anything.

I hope that all the people could be relieved of the pain and live a relaxed life.

Conquer the incurable pain

Mr Kikuchyo Kanagawa County jobless 70

In the intense competition in the modern society of communication, I caught duodenal ulcer at the age of 58. After retirement, I caught herpes zoster at the age of 68 and suffered a lot from intercostal neuralgia. A friend of mine who used to suffer from the same symptom suggested me receiving treatment at hospital immediately. Since the condition of my family did not allow, I often woke up at midnight for the great pain.

During this time, acupuncture and moxibustion treatment eliminated the pimple and red on the skin, but intercostal neuralgia still remained. Afterwards, my strength declined, I felt weak in back and feet and cold in my limbs. I thought I was going to die. Later I thought that "a sound digestive system is the basic of health", so I began to search among traditional Chinese medicines available in Japan for suitable medicine for digestive system. It happened that I came to know the natural nutritious liquid at doctor Wang Zhengguo's speech. I began to drink it immediately and exciting effect was achieved!

Marvelous effect made me excited!

It tastes sour and sweet as if I had drunk it before, and I have really felt its effect on digestive organs. I pick up confidence in health although I am physically weakened. The natural nutritious liquid not only works on digestive organs, warm my hands and feet, but also has anti-cancer function. So in my opinion, traditional Chinese medicine helps recover the function of internal organs.

I am now in late seventies. Combining western and Chinese medicine, it seems as if the natural nutritious liquid were bestowed by God. Here I'd like to express my gratitude again.

Patient of Iron-deficiency Anemia enjoying delicious food again

Mr Nohara Tokyo employee of a company 39

It is twenty years since I was found to have anaemia in a blood test. To be specific, it is iron-deficiency anemia. Sometimes the disease got serious so that I had to receive blood transfusion. Besides, I was hospitalized for one year for blood transfusion caused acute hepatitis. Fortunately, I did not feel typical symptoms of anaemia such as daze. And even when I caught hepatitis, I did not lose appetite, nor had jaundice.

Soon afterwards, my liver function returned to normal. My white blood cells, red blood cells and haemoglobin maintained on low levels. So I began to try various health foods. Although I ate rough rice food, my blood circulation was still not good. My body couldn't take in nutrition and there was no sign of improvement. My weight did not rise and I remained physically weak like before.

Four or five years ago, I resumed yoga which was suspended for some time and I grew stronger little by little. At that time, I began to drink the natural nutritious liquid I had heard of. The list of ingredients shows that a bottle of 10ml natural nutritious liquid contains such natural medicinal herbs as ginseng, Chinese caterpillar fungus, glossy ganoderma, etc, each of which has unique function. Besides, since it also contains honey, it tastes sweet and is easy to drink.

Every time I drank the natural nutritious liquid before meal, I had appetite. I couldn't drink a large amount of water at one time in usual times, but I could drink the natural nutritious liquid easily three times a day, in the morning, at

353

noon and at night. The health examination three months later showed that red blood cells, white blood cells, haemoglobin and blood cell specific volumn were within the normal range. All my friends and relatives were surprised and glad at my rising weight.

Everyone has different way of keeping healthy. As for me, the natural nutritious liquid and yoga are most suitable for me. I'm so happy to find the suitable way to keep healthy. I'll continue in this way.

Natural nutritious liquid removes daze

Miss Sakara Tokyo employee of a company 29

In this year, I often felt dazed and was easy to get tired. Even my heartbeat quickened. But I was physically weak from childhood and I suffered a lot from dysmenorrhoea, so I did not take it seriously. However, these symptoms aggravated, so I went to the ear-nose-throat section, eye section and obstetrics section for examination, and the results were invariably "???abnormal, exhausted, anaemia", which made me depressed. I had no choice but to take medicines.

But there was no sign of improvement and even my sense of taste became strange. Roast meat is my favorite but I could not swallow a small piece. My weight began to drop. When I was spending every day, dazed, I got to know doctor Wang Zhengguo, who came to Japan to deliver a speech.

At first sight of me, doctor Wang said, "your physical state is so bad. It may be due to the weakening function of thyroid gland." It pointed to the problem. I immediately accepted doctor Wang's suggestion to take the natural nutritious liquid. On the first day, I felt energetic. It is so marvelous.

Before that, the dog (female, 40kg) that belonged to my family had a cancer on her gingiva and it grew bigger. After an operation was performed to cut it off, the doctor said "it is sure to attack again." Just as expected, the tumor at this part grew even bigger. All my family did not have the heart to see her suffer so much. I thought the medicine that works on people must have the same effect on animals. So I also placed an order for Tian Xian liquid and let her drink eight bottles of it per day and I poured Tian Xian liquid on a clean rag and applied it to the affected part. Seeing her so joyous, I believed that it was the natural instinct of animals. As a result, the tumor grew smaller and disappeared completely four months later!

After this experience, I began to drink two bottles of the natural nutritious liquid per day.

Two weeks later, since there wasn't much change to my body, I thought of giving it up. But eventually I went on. My appetite began to recover from the third week and my mental and physical state returned to normal gradually. Finally, the daze that had troubled me disappeared. Only the person concerned could feel the experiences. I don't have to take other medicines any more. And my rough skin gradually becomes soft.

It is three months since I began to drink the natural nutritious liquid. My weight has recovered and I can enjoy the delicious roast meat again. Since I haven't tasted it for long, I eat a lot. Now I am faced with another problem --- overweight.